# Tai Chi Chin Na

THE SEIZING ART OF TAI CHI CHUAN

太極擒拿

法然

# DR. YANG, JWING-MING

# Tai Chi Chin Na

## THE SEIZING ART OF TAI CHI CHUAN

YMAA Publication Center, Inc.
Wolfeboro, NH USA

**YMAA Publication Center, Inc.**
PO Box 480
Wolfeboro, NH 03894
800 669-8892 • www.ymaa.com • info@ymaa.com

ISBN: 9781594393075 (Print) • 9781594393082 (Ebook)

Second edition copyright ©1995, 2014 by Dr. Yang, Jwing-Ming
Cover design and anatomy image enhancements by Axie Breen
Copyedit by Dolores Sparrow and T. G. LaFredo
Caption editing by Leslie Takao
Proofreading by Sara Scanlon
Index by Dolores Sparrow
Photos by YMAA unless noted otherwise, Ramel Rones was the photograph model.
This book has been typeset in Adobe Garamond and Trade Gothic and printed on #60 FSC Husky Offset.

Original anatomy images copyright ©1994 by TechPool Studios Corp. USA, 1463 Warrensville Center Road, Cleveland, OH 44121.

POD 1216

### Publisher's Cataloging in Publication

Yang, Jwing-Ming, 1946-

Tai chi chin na : the seizing art of tai chi chuan / Dr. Yang, Jwing-Ming. -- 2nd ed. -- Wolfeboro, NH USA : YMAA Publication Center, [2014]

    pages ; cm.

    ISBN: 978-1-59439-307-5 (print) ; 978-1-59439-308-2 (ebook)
    Revised edition of: Taiji chin na (qin na). YMAA, c1995.
    Includes bibliography and index.
    Summary: Tai chi chin na will help you include martial art grappling skills in your tai chi training. This book provides a solid and practical approach to learning specific techniques that flow from each movement, the proper hand forms to use when striking or pressing cavities, and the locations for targeting cavities on the body.--Publisher.

    1. Tai chi. 2. Martial arts--Training. 3. Hand-to-hand fighting, Oriental--Training. 4. Self-defense. 5. Kung fu. 6. Qi gong. 7. Martial arts--Psychological aspects. I. Title. II. Taiji chin na (qin na).

GV504 .Y37 2014                       2014949077

613.7/148--dc23                   1410

# Dedication

To my first tai chi teacher
Kao Tao

謹奉獻給高濤老師

Proverbs

*"The taller the bamboo grows, the lower it bows."*
*"The truly humble always know others, and do not care if other people know them."*
*"Those who have to criticize others are those whose minds are void."*
*"The yin side of dignity is false pride and self-spite."*
*"Those who despise themselves are always concerned with their dignity."*

# Editorial Notes

## Romanization of Chinese Words

The interior of this book primarily uses the Pinyin romanization system of Chinese to English. In some instances, a more popular word may be used as an aid for reader convenience, such as "tai chi" in place of the Pinyin spelling, taiji. Pinyin is standard in the People's Republic of China and in several world organizations, including the United Nations. Pinyin, which was introduced in China in the 1950s, replaces the older Wade-Giles and Yale systems.

Some common conversions are found in the following:

| Pinyin | Also spelled as | Pronunciation |
| --- | --- | --- |
| qi | chi | chē |
| qigong | chi kung | chē gōng |
| qin na | chin na | chǐn nǎ |
| jing | jin | jǐn |
| gongfu | kung fu | gōng foo |
| taijiquan | tai chi chuan | tī jē chǔén |

For more information, please refer to *The People's Republic of China: Administrative Atlas*; *The Reform of the Chinese Written Language*; or a contemporary manual of style.

## Formats and Treatment of Chinese Words

The first instances of foreign words in the text proper are set in italics whenever possible. For readability, the Pinyin term "an" is italicized throughout: "*an*."

Transliterations are provided frequently: for example, Eight Pieces of Brocade (*Ba Duan Jin*, 八段錦).

Chinese persons' names are mostly presented in their more popular English spelling. Capitalization is according to the *Chicago Manual of Style* 16th edition. The author or publisher may use a specific spelling or capitalization in respect to the living or deceased person. For example, Cheng, Man-ch'ing can be written as Zheng Manqing.

## Photographs

Many photographs include motion arrows to help show the starting position of the body motion.

# Table of Contents

# Foreword by Grandmaster Li, Mao-Ching

The origin of *taiji* (太極) is misty and turbid; we call it *wuji* (無極) (no extremity). When it is extremely calm, it appears condensed and peaceful externally. However, concealed within it there exists both *yin* (陰) and *yang* (陽). These two, yin and yang, mutually transport, vary, advance, and withdraw. Consequently, there is neither void nor defect. The name we give to this hidden movement of yin and yang is "taiji."

Application of this theory to two-person taiji pushing hands practice reveals the same twin virtues of yin and yang. You and your partner mutually harmonize and coordinate with each other, and thereby improve both your own and each other's health. Taiji is used not only for defensive purposes. It says in the *Yi Jing*, or *Book of Changes* (易經), that "the [hidden] beginning of the misty origin [i.e., wuji] is called taiji. From the nourishment of the two poles [i.e., yin and yang], ten thousand objects were born."[1]

The word "taiji" was first seen in the *Yi Jing*. Though the word "taiji" was also mentioned in the *Han Book*, it recognized that this word originated from the *Yi Jing*. In the *Yi Jing*, it says, "Taiji is the key which dominates the generations and variations. [It] is the mother of the million objects between heaven and earth. [If we] trace the beginning of the world, it is certain that it originated from this—the sole misty qi." It also says, "Taiji, the master of the qi, is the order [i.e., rule] and the great foundation of the generations and variations is the origin of the sole qi. Therefore, it is called 'the grand ultimate.' Fu Xi saw taiji as the dawn of the day. It is the mother of the beginning. The origin of the million [objects] and the source of the sole qi, therefore, is called 'grand ultimate,' [which is] able to generate, originate, and transport without stop."[2, 3]

It is said, "Knowing the origin, it is easy to figure out the root. Consequently, it is easy to explore the branches and leaves."[4] Therefore, the ultimate holy man (Confucius) said, "The gentleman keeps the origin. When the origin is firmly established, the Dao can then be begotten."[5] This is to encourage people. It means that the importance of education is in its origin. Taiji is the mother of the million objects between heaven and earth. This origin from taiji begets countless generations. All of these vary from the sole qi. That is why heaven and earth also reside within taiji and are able to move ceaselessly. The birth of taiji is the origin of the beginning. When this origin is applied to humanity, it is called original qi.

The million objects originated from original qi. It then derived into yin and yang, and followed with the four natural variations of the seasons. From this, we can see that qi is the mother of the million objects. Therefore, when a human wishes to strengthen the body, he must first regulate the qi. If the qi is smooth and uniform, then the foundation of health can be established. This is the real meaning of variation in taiji.

Among the five internal yin organs in the human body, the kidneys acquire the prebirth qi. This prebirth qi is also called original qi or the real qi. The stomach area (middle *dan tian*) stores the postbirth qi. In order to establish smooth and uniform qi, a healthy condition of the kidneys and stomach is the main goal of qigong practice.

Externally, you should train the fist techniques, and internally you should cultivate and regulate the qi to nourish life. When qi is circulated smoothly, then the muscles/tendons (physical body) will be comfortable and the blood circulation can be free. Naturally, hundreds of sicknesses will not occur.

When we apply taiji into the origins of humanity, it is like a miniature heaven and earth. Before it is discriminated, it is calmness. Once it is divided, then yin and yang are discriminated (i.e., male and female). When this yin and yang are manifest in this world, the four seasons are derived and the five elements of qi are generated. These five qi are metal, wood, water, fire, and dust. When these five qi are applied to humanity, they correspond to the lungs, liver, kidneys, heart, and spleen, which are the five yin internal organs. These five qi can also be applied to the east, west, south, north, and center.

The five elements have natural patterns of mutual generation and conquest following yin and yang theory. From the patterns of the five elements and the theory of yin and yang, millions of lives are derived and endure. When these patterns and theories are applied to the human body, it can become very strong. Among all of the Chinese martial arts, taijiquan holds the first place, for it carries these five patterns and yin and yang theory. Therefore, a taijiquan practitioner's ability to reach a profound level depends on how much he is able to ponder and understand the above theory.

When taijiquan is practiced, it is as soft as the falling leaves blown by autumn wind. But internally, it is storing the yang and can assume shape as a sharp sword that is able to cut the vine and branches easily. The theory is simple, because you must know how to be relaxed, and then be able to tense at the correct instant. When you are relaxed, your mind is calm, neutral, and empty, until you feel you are transparent and invisible. It is like clouds at dawn or dusk, peaceful, calm, and utterly still. Once the stored jing is manifested, it is like a hurricane whirlwind, fast and powerful.

If a taijiquan practitioner understands the theory of yin and yang, and the mutual relations of the five elements, then he can be calm and round. He can also be strong internally, and manifest strength externally. Naturally, the means of reaching this goal are through ceaseless study and practice.

When taijiquan is applied externally, it is manifested into the four fighting categories: kicking (*ti*, 踢), striking (*da*, 打), wrestling (*shuai*, 摔), and seize and control (*na*, 拿). This book will introduce the applications of qin na in taijiquan.

The two words "qin na" were first used by the Zejiang Police Academy before World War II, in 1937. At that time, the principal of this academy, Mr. Zhao, Long-wen (趙龍文) was known as an excellent scholar. He was also a lover and promoter of the Chinese martial arts. At that time, all of the students, male or female, were required to learn and practice qin na, wrestling, and defense against both the dagger and the gun. The teacher was Mr. Han, Ching-tang (韓慶堂), and the assistants were Mrs. Jiang, Tang-zhu (江溏珠) and her husband. Mrs. Jiang was the daughter of a well-known retired Qing martial officer at that time. Later, Mr. Han's martial arts brother, Mr. Liu, Jin-sheng (劉錦昇), was also appointed as a coach, in order to satisfy the great demand for teaching. When they had time, they got together and mutually studied the techniques of dividing the muscle/tendon and misplacing the bone (分筋搓骨手法). If they felt less than smooth or had difficulty, they would ask for the answer from Mrs. Jiang's father. From these efforts, they compiled a complete record of the postures used both in solo practice and also in mutual matching qin na. This compilation was then named the *Police Qin Na Applications* (分筋搓骨手法), or simply *Qin Na Techniques* (擒拿術). All of this history has been recounted in Dr. Yang's book *Comprehensive Applications of Shaolin Chin Na*. I will not repeat it here. I will only conclude this foreword with some of the important points for qin na applications, and the requirements of success. This will enable you to reach a stage of "applying the techniques as you wish" (順心應手) and achieve effective control of your opponent. From my accumulation of more than fifty years of martial arts experience, I understand that a practitioner must have a firm foundation in Chinese gongfu. Only then can he unify body and hands. Under these conditions, his legs will be able to coordinate the techniques naturally and smoothly. This is the key to winning and making the techniques effective.

Qin na and taiji have close relations that cannot be separated. When qin na is applied into the eight trigrams derived from taiji, it occupies the word "thunder" (雷). This has the meaning of "thunder" in the eight trigrams. Among all taijiquan techniques, pluck (*cai*, 採), pulling (*le*, 将), capture (*lu*, 擄), press down (*an*, 按), elbow (*zhou*, 肘), and bump (*kao*, 靠) are commonly adopted in qin na. When qin na is applied in taijiquan, the defensive theory remains the same, using the soft against the hard. The only difference is that once qin na is used to lock the opponent in position, the final control must be firm and hard. Though the result is different, the original theory remains the same.

When a practitioner learns Chinese gongfu (which implies external styles) and has a strong foundation, then he will be able to unify the hands, eyes (i.e., reaction), body (i.e., movements), techniques, and stepping (手、眼、身、法、步). This will let you reach a stage of emitting power from the hands with speed like thunder, which does not allow anyone time to cover his ears. You attack the opponent without his expectation or preparation. In addition, you will be able to maneuver your strategies and vary your plan as you wish. In this case, you will have an advantage in catching the right timing and emitting your thunder strength. But remember: Once you are delayed, you will have lost the opportunity. In taiji, it is said, "One movement, ten thousand variations."

Again, I am very happy to hear that Dr. Yang, Jwing-Ming has completed this book, *Tai Chi Chin Na*, to share his knowledge with the public. I am so delighted that I have summarized the lessons and experience I have accumulated from my teacher about qin na. This can be used for your reference.

Li, Mao-Ching (李茂清)
Research Member
Guoshu Promoting Committee
Republic of China
February 15, 1995

## References

1. 易："渾元之始，是曰太極。二象所資，萬品之所生。"（孔子家語）
2. 易註："太極者，主生化之樞，為天地萬物之母，而溯世界之初始，則固來之，渾然一氣也。"；"太極者，氣之主宰，其生化之序，生成變化之大本，一氣之源也，故曰太極。"；"伏羲之一畫，即太極，為一體，是太初之母，萬有之宗，一氣之源，故曰太極，能生，有始，運行不息。"（伏羲）
3. Fu Xi was the Chinese emperor during the legendary period (2852–2737 BC).
4. 易經："所謂知其源，則流易測得其本，則枝葉易探。"
5. 聖曰："君子務本，本立而道生。"

# Foreword by Grandmaster Jou, Tsung-Hwa

After finishing this book, Master Yang, Jwing-Ming shared it with me. I feel that this book is of great quality and I would like to offer some words about it.

First of all, this book is written by a very credible author, because Dr. Yang has a very high level of education in the Chinese martial arts. Most Chinese martial artists only have a background in either theory or practice, but Dr. Yang has a solid background in both. He also has a high level of Western education, having graduated with a PhD from Purdue University. He exhibits a fervent desire to share the wonders of Chinese martial arts with westerners, and his broad background in both Eastern and Western knowledge makes him a fine teacher.

Traditional *chin na* (*qin na*) books are mostly theoretical in nature, which makes learning from them difficult and incomplete. But because Dr. Yang makes such explicit use of pictures to show the techniques of chin na step by step, this book serves very well as a self-teaching guide. Also, because of his popular YMAA schools, and his many worldwide workshops, this book makes a fine lesson accompaniment as well, especially for those who find it otherwise difficult to learn by books alone.

I am sure readers will find this chin na book informative as well as interesting.

Jou, Tsung-Hwa (周宗樺)
(July 13, 1917–August 3, 1998)
January 12, 1995

# Foreword by Master Liang, Shou-Yu

I am very happy to see this book, *Tai Chi Chin Na*, available in publication. This again is a great contribution made by Dr. Yang to the world martial arts society. He has constantly introduced and contributed the knowledge he has obtained from Chinese culture and from his personal intelligent study and research. This kind of spirit is precious and difficult to find.

The contents of *taijiquan* are very wide and profound. People always know that *taiji* can maintain health, strengthen the physical and qi bodies, relax the mind and spirit, cultivate an individual's personality, and regulate the emotional and wisdom minds. However, many people are not aware that it can also offer a practitioner a great foundation for self-defense. From the drills of pushing hands and taiji sparring, a practitioner is able to comprehend the keys of leading *jing* (*yin jing*, 引勁), neutralizing jing (*hua jing*, 化勁), coiling jing (*chan jing*, 纏勁), emitting jing (*fa jing*, 發勁), understanding jing (*dong jing*, 懂勁), and many other skills for using the soft against the hard.

To Chinese martial arts society, taijiquan is a widely accepted martial skill that can be used for health and self-defense. It contains the four required fighting skills and categories: kicking (*ti*, 踢), striking (*da*, 打), wrestling (*shuai*, 摔), and *qin na* (*na*, 拿). This book, *Tai Chi Chin Na*, introduces the correct and accurate qin na applications and tricks that can be used in the taiji eight basic technical patterns or jing: wardoff (*peng*, 掤), rollback (*lu*, 掘), press or squeeze (*ji*, 擠), press or push down (*an*, 按), pluck (*cai*, 採), rend or split (*lie*, 挒), elbow (*zhou*, 肘), and lean or press against (*kao*, 靠). This book also introduces the qin na applications that can be applied from the thirty-seven basic taijiquan movements. Although taijiquan develops many qin na skills, there has never been anyone who could compile and introduce them to the general public.

Dr. Yang has performed deep research in qin na. His knowledge is the widest and the most profound among those qin na experts whom I have known. He has written many other qin na books; all have been widely welcomed and appreciated. He has introduced and shared his many years of personal taiji and qin na experience to Western martial society. To the best of my knowledge, this is the first written book on taiji qin na available in the world. I deeply believe that the publication of this book will enable readers to enhance their understanding of how to apply qin na in taijiquan.

Liang, Shou-Yu (梁守渝)
Vancouver, Canada
December 1, 1994

# Preface by Dr. Yang, Jwing-Ming

Even though *qin na* (*chin na*) has been popularly practiced in Chinese martial arts for hundreds of years, it was not until the 1982 publication of my first qin na book, *Shaolin Chin Na*, by Unique Publications, that these secret techniques of the Chinese martial arts were widely revealed to the Western world. Since then, this art has grown so rapidly that my book has been translated into several different languages, making its way all over the world in less than ten years.

Later, due to the tremendous number of requests, I decided to write another volume to discuss qin na theory and techniques in a more in-depth manner. Therefore, the second volume, *The Analysis of Shaolin Chin Na*, was published in 1987 by YMAA. It is beyond my belief that in such a short time, this art has grown so wide and popular that I have to travel to more than thirteen countries around the world at least twice a year to teach this art. I believe that the main reason for this is simply because this art can be adopted easily by almost all martial arts styles and blended into their own techniques. In addition to this, the qin na art has been proven to be one of the most effective defensive techniques, and it can be learned easily, even by a martial arts beginner.

From my experience teaching seminars, I realize that the hardest aspect of the art is not learning the techniques themselves, but applying those techniques to dynamic situations. Usually, a practitioner can pick up a technique easily and make it effective only when his partner is cooperative. However, as we already know, when you encounter an enemy in real life, his cooperation is unlikely. Any success in executing a technique depends on how accurate, fast, natural, and automatic your reactions are, and the only way to develop skills in these areas is to practice. For this reason, I decided to write my third qin na book, *Comprehensive Applications of Shaolin Chin Na*, published by YMAA, 1994, making this "seizing and controlling" art more complete.

As is well known in Chinese martial arts society, qin na techniques have been an integral part of every Chinese martial art style. It is not like Japanese jujitsu, which is considered a style in itself. It is my understanding that there is no known "qin na style" in Chinese martial arts. The reason for this is very simple. It is well known that there are four main fighting categories in every Chinese martial style. These four categories are striking by hands (*da*, 打), kicking with legs (*ti*, 踢), wrestling (*shuai*, 摔), and seize and control (*na*, 拿). It is also a fact that a substantial portion of Japanese culture was imported from China, beginning in the Chinese Han dynasty (206 BC–AD 221). It is further believed that the martial techniques that exist in Japan have been heavily influenced by the Chinese martial arts. When striking and kicking techniques passed to Japan and became karate styles, Chinese wrestling became judo, and qin na techniques were transformed into the art of jujitsu. Many Japanese martial artists believe that the aikido martial arts were actually developed from the theories of Chinese *taijiquan* and qin na. From this you can see why qin na is not, in itself, considered a style in China.

There are also many qin na techniques in taijiquan. In fact, due to the emphasis on sticking and adhering techniques in taijiquan's close-range fighting strategy, qin na techniques have always been a very important part of the art. In this book, I will try my best to introduce to the reader those qin na techniques that I know can be applied into taijiquan fighting. In truth, many of these techniques actually originated in my White Crane Style. The reason that I can apply White Crane Qin Na into taijiquan easily is very simple. Taijiquan is known as a soft style and White Crane as a soft-hard style. It does not matter externally; the theory behind the soft side of White Crane remains the same as that of taijiquan. Many nonproficient Chinese martial artists believe that if taijiquan is interpreted by another style's theory or its theories have been blended with another style, then it is not pure taijiquan. They do not know that taijiquan actually originated from Shaolin styles, and therefore it was built and evolved over the same theoretical root. For example, it is well known that the first routine of Chen Style Taijiquan is called *changquan* (長拳) (long fist) and the second routine, called *pao chui* (炮捶) (cannon fist), all originated from the Shaolin Temple. In fact, from a historical perspective, those profound taiji masters of the past are all known to have learned many other different styles. For example, Sun, Lu-tang (孫祿堂), Zhang, Zhao-dong (張兆東), Wang, Shu-tian (王樹田), Han, Ching-tang (韓慶堂), and many others were all experts in many different styles. The Chinese martial arts grew and developed in the same cultural environment as the yin and yang theory. From learning different styles, you are afforded different angles of viewing the same techniques. This is the way of Dao.

Finally, you should understand one important fact: like many other Chinese martial arts, though a great portion of basic qin na techniques can simply be learned from books and videos, very often a qualified master is still necessary to lead you to a profound level. Books can offer you the theory of the techniques, while videos can offer you the continuous movements of the techniques. However, neither of these two can offer you the correct feeling of the locking and a clear concept of how an angle is set up. Because of this, if you are sincere in becoming a proficient qin na expert, you should also participate in seminars offered by qualified qin na masters. Very often, only a few minutes in a qin na seminar can solve the confusion and questions that might have taken you months or even years to figure out.

Other than merely reading this book, an interested reader should refer to the book *Shaolin Chin Na*, published by Unique Publications, as well as *Analysis of Shaolin Chin Na* and *Comprehensive Applications of Shaolin Chin Na*, published by YMAA. These three books will help you build a firm foundation, both in theory and in routine practice. In addition, these three books—especially the second one—will teach you how to train the power required for qin na techniques and the theory and methods of how to treat common injuries. In the appendix of the second volume, some secret herbal prescriptions for injuries, taught to me by my White Crane master, are also included. In order to avoid replication, we will not repeat these subjects in this volume.

In this volume, you may notice that all of the Chinese pronunciations are spelled according to the Pinyin system. The reason for this is simply that the Pinyin system has become more popular than any other system in the last fifteen years. It is believed that this system will become the most common and popular system in the next few decades.

Dr. Yang, Jwing-Ming (楊俊敏)
January, 1995

# Chapter 1: General Concepts

## 1-1. Introduction

*Taijiquan* (太極拳) was originally developed for combat in ancient times. Its fighting theory is to use the soft against the hard, and to use the round to neutralize the straight or square. In order to achieve this goal, the body must be soft and the movements must be smooth and natural. Taijiquan also emphasizes the cultivation of *qi* (氣), or internal energy. The concentrated mind leads the qi to circulate in the body. Because of this, taijiquan can be used for maintaining health and improving longevity.

Because of its effectiveness, since the 1940s, taijiquan has become publicly accepted as one of the best *qigong* (氣功) practices for health. Unfortunately, due to the overemphasis of its health aspects, the essence of taijiquan's creation—martial applications—has gradually been ignored. It is very upsetting to see that, even in modern China, most taijiquan practitioners do not understand this martial essence of taijiquan. Naturally, they do not understand martial power (*jing*, 勁) and the theory of using the mind to lead the qi to energize muscular power to its maximum. Consequently, the martial applications of each movement have begun to slowly disappear.

In order to make the art of taijiquan complete, I believe that it is our obligation to again study its martial applications. Only from this study will we be able to recover its lost essence and find the root of its creation. Only then can its health benefits be completely comprehended. In this book, one type of taijiquan martial applications, *qin na* (擒拿), will be introduced to you. I hope that through this introduction, general taijiquan practitioners will be inspired and encouraged to discuss and find the real essence of their art.

### What is Qin Na?

"Qin" (chin) (擒) in Chinese means "to seize or catch," in the way an eagle seizes a rabbit or a policeman "catches a murderer" (*qin xiong*, 擒兇). "Na" (拿) means "to hold and control." Therefore, qin na can be translated as "seize and control."

Generally speaking, in order to have effective and efficient fighting capability, almost all Chinese martial styles include four categories of techniques. The first category is composed of the techniques of striking, punching, pushing, pressing, etc. The second category is using the leg to kick, sweep, step, or trip. In these techniques, contact time between you and your opponent must be very short, and the power for attacking is usually explosive and harmful. The third category is called wrestling (*shuai jiao*, 摔跤), and it contains the skills of destroying the opponent's root and balance, consequently throwing him down. Often these techniques are mixed with the leg's sweeping or tripping, and the body's swinging or even throwing. The last category is qin na, containing grabbing techniques that specialize in controlling or locking the opponent's joints, muscles, or tendons.

However, you should understand an important fact. In a combat situation, the above three categories are often applied together, and cannot really be separated. For example, while one of your hands is grabbing and controlling your opponent, the other hand is used to strike a vital cavity. Another example of this is that often you use grabbing to lock your opponent's joints while throwing him down for further attack. Because of this, sometimes it is very difficult to discriminate clearly between techniques in a real situation. As a matter of fact, many Chinese martial artists believe that since there are many other non-grabbing techniques, such as pressing or striking the cavities or nerves, which can make the opponent numb in part of the body (or even render him unconscious), thereby providing control of the opponent, these techniques should also be recognized as qin na. You can see that, as long as the techniques are able to immobilize an opponent, it does not matter if the cause is a joint lock, numbness, or unconsciousness—all of them can be classified as qin na.

In summary, grabbing qin na techniques control and lock the opponent's joints or muscles/tendons so he cannot move, thus neutralizing his fighting ability. Pressing qin na techniques are used to numb the opponent's limbs, causing him to lose consciousness, or even die. Pressing qin na is usually applied to the qi cavities to disrupt normal qi circulation to the organs or the brain. Pressing techniques are also frequently used on nerve endings to cause extreme pain and unconsciousness. Qin na striking techniques are applied to vital points, and can be very deadly. Cavities on the qi channels can be attacked, or certain vital areas struck to rupture arteries. All of these techniques serve to "seize and control" the opponent. Therefore, qin na techniques can be generally categorized as follows:[1]

1. Dividing the muscle/tendon (*fen jin*, 分筋)
2. Misplacing the bone (*cuo gu*, 錯骨)
3. Sealing the breath (*bi qi*, 閉氣)
4. Pressing a vein/artery (*dian mai*, 點脈) or sealing or blocking the vein/artery (*duan mai*, 斷脈)[2]
5. Cavity press (*dian xue*, 點穴) or pressing a primary qi channel (*dian mai*, 點脈)[3]

Within these categories, fen jin also includes grabbing the muscle/tendon (*zhua jin*, 抓筋), and dian xue also includes grabbing or pressing the cavities (*na xue*, 拿穴).

Generally, dividing the muscle/tendon, misplacing the bone, and some techniques of sealing the breath are relatively easy to learn, and the theory behind them is easy to understand. They usually require only muscular strength and practice to make the control effective. When these same techniques are used to break bones or injure joints or tendons, you usually need to use martial power (jing, 勁). (For a discussion of jing, see the author's book *Tai Chi Theory and Martial Power,* published by YMAA.) Sealing the vein/artery and pressing the cavities require detailed knowledge of the location and depth of the cavities, the timing of the qi circulation, development of mind (*yi*, 意), internal energy (qi, 氣), martial power (jing, 勁), and special hand forms and techniques. This usually requires formal instruction by a qualified master, not only because the knowledge is deep, but also because most of the techniques are learned from sensing and feeling. Many of the techniques can easily cause death, and for this reason a master will normally only pass down this knowledge to students who are moral and trustworthy.

## Qin Na in Chinese Martial Arts

Nobody can tell exactly when qin na was first used. It probably began the first time one person grabbed another with the intention of controlling him. Grabbing the opponent's limbs or weapon is one of the most basic and instinctive means of immobilizing him or controlling his actions.

Because of their practicality, qin na techniques have been trained right along with other fighting techniques since the beginning of Chinese martial arts, many thousands of years ago. Although no system has sprung up that practices only qin na, almost every martial style has qin na mixed in with its other techniques. Even in Japan, Korea, and other Oriental countries that have been significantly influenced by Chinese culture, the indigenous martial styles have qin na techniques mixed in to some degree.

Generally speaking, since martial styles in southern China specialize in hand techniques and close-range fighting, they tend to have better-developed qin na techniques, and they tend to rely more upon them than do the northern styles. Also, because southern martial styles emphasize hand conditioning more than the northern styles, they tend to use more muscles for grabbing and cavity press. Southern styles' emphasis on short-range fighting causes them to train more for sticking and adhering. The techniques are usually applied with a circular motion, which can set up the opponent for a qin na control without his feeling the preparation. Footwork is also considered a very important part of qin na training for a southern martial artist. Remember that these statements are only generalizations; there are northern styles that also emphasize these things.

In Chinese internal styles, such as *taiji* (太極) and liu he ba fa (六合八法), neutralization is usually done with a circular motion, and so the qin na techniques tend to be smooth and round. Often the opponent will be controlled before he realizes that a technique is being applied. In coordination with circular stepping, circular qin na can be used to pull the opponent's root and throw him away.

Japanese jujitsu and aikido are based on the same principles as qin na and taiji. Since these countries were significantly influenced by Chinese culture, it seems probable that Chinese qin na also influenced their indigenous martial arts.

Since fundamental qin na techniques can be used to seize and control a criminal without injuring or killing him, they have been an important part of training for constables, government officers, and modern policemen. Around AD 527, the Shaolin Temple (少林寺) became heavily involved in the martial arts. Since many nonlethal qin na techniques are very effective, the martial artists at the temple extensively researched, developed, and trained them. In the late Qing dynasty (清朝) in the nineteenth century, Shaolin techniques were taught to people in the general population, and qin na techniques were passed down along with the different martial styles that were developed in the Shaolin Temple. Many qin na techniques were also developed for use with weapons specially designed to seize the opponent's weapon. If your opponent is disarmed, he is automatically in a disadvantageous situation. For example, the hook of the hook sword and the hand guard of a *chai* (*sai*) (釵) were designed for this purpose.

## 1-2. Qin Na Categories and Theory

Although qin na techniques from one gongfu style may seem quite different from the techniques of another style, the theories and principles of application remain the same. These theories and principles form the root of all qin na techniques. If you adhere to these roots, your qin na will continue to grow and improve, but if you ignore these roots, your qin na will always remain undeveloped. In this section we will discuss these general theories and principles.

Before we discuss each qin na category, you should understand that there is no technique that is perfect for all situations. What you do depends upon what your opponent does, and since your opponent will not stand still and just let you control him, you must be able to adapt your qin na to fit the circumstances. Like all martial arts techniques, your qin na must respond to and follow the situation; techniques must be skillful, alive, fast, and powerful. You should further understand that qin na must take the opponent by surprise. In grabbing qin na you have to grasp your opponent's body, and so if your opponent is aware of your intention, it will be extremely difficult for you to successfully apply the technique. In such a case you may be obliged to use a cavity strike qin na instead of a grabbing technique.

It is usually much easier to strike the opponent than to control him. Subduing an opponent through a qin na controlling technique is a way to show mercy to someone you do not want to injure. To successfully apply a grabbing qin na, you often need to fake or strike the opponent first to set him up for your controlling technique. For example, you can use a punch to cause your opponent to block, and when he blocks, you quickly grab his hand and use qin na to control him. Alternatively, you might kick his shin first to draw his attention to his leg, and immediately grab his hand and control him.

As mentioned, there are five categories of qin na:

1. Dividing the muscle/tendon or grabbing the muscle/tendon (fen jin or zhua jin, 分筋 / 抓筋)

2. Misplacing the bone (cuo gu, 錯骨)

3. Sealing the breath (bi qi, 閉氣)

4. Vein/artery press or sealing the vein/artery (dian mai or duan mai, 點脈 / 斷脈)

5. Pressing primary qi channel or cavity press (dian mai or dian xue, 點脈 / 點穴)

This book will discuss all of these categories in detail except the last two, which will be discussed only on an introductory level because they require an in-depth understanding of qi circulation, acupuncture, and specialized training techniques.

One additional point needs to be mentioned here. Very often qin na techniques make use of principles from several categories at once. For example, many techniques simultaneously use the principles of dividing the muscle/tendon and misplacing the bone.

## 1. Fen Jin or Zhua Jin (分筋 / 抓筋) (Dividing the Muscle/Tendon or Grabbing the Muscle/Tendon)

"Fen" (分) in Chinese means "to divide," "zhua" (抓) means "to grab," and "jin" (筋) means "tendon, sinew, or muscle." Fen jin or zhua jin qin na refers to techniques that tear apart the opponent's muscles or tendons. Muscles contain nerves and many qi branch channels, so when you tear a muscle or tendon, not only do you cause sensations of pain to travel to the brain, but you also directly or indirectly affect the qi and interfere with the normal functioning of the organs. If the pain is great enough, it can disturb the qi and seriously damage the organs, and in extreme cases can even cause death. For this reason, when you are in extreme pain, your brain may "give the order" for you to pass out. Once you are unconscious, the qi circulation will significantly decrease, which will limit damage to the organs and perhaps save your life.

Fen jin qin na uses two main methods to divide the muscle/tendon. One method is to twist the opponent's joint and then bend. Twisting the joint also twists the muscles/tendons. If you bend the joint at the same time, you can tear the tendons off the bone.

The second method is to split and tear the muscle/tendon apart without twisting. The most common place to do this is the fingers.

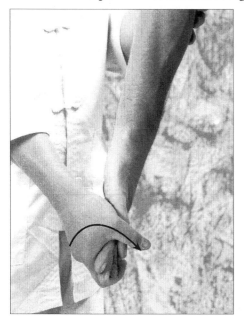

Method 1: Twist the joint.

Then bend the fingers.

Method 2: Split and tear the muscle/tendon without twisting.

Grabbing the muscle/tendon (zhua jin) relies upon the strength of the fingers to grab, press, and then pull the opponent's large muscles or tendons. This causes pain by overextending the muscles and tendons. Common targets for zhua jin qin na are the tendon on the shoulder, under the armpit, on the neck, and on the sides of the waist. Zhua jin qin na is used particularly by the Eagle Claw and Tiger Claw Styles. Although zhua jin is usually classified with fen jin qin na, many Chinese martial artists separate the two categories because the principle used to divide the muscle/tendon is different.

Grabbing the muscle/tendon at the shoulder.

Grabbing the muscle/tendon at the armpit front side.

Grabbing the muscle/tendon at the armpit rear side.

Grabbing the muscle/tendon at the neck.

Grabbing the muscle/tendon at the side of the waist.

### 2. Cuo Gu (錯骨) (Misplacing the Bone)

"Cuo" (錯) means "wrong, disorder, or to place wrongly," and "gu" (骨) means "bone." Cuo gu, therefore, are qin na techniques that put bones in the wrong positions. These techniques are usually applied to the joints. If you examine the structure of a joint, you will see that the bones are connected to each other by ligaments, and the muscles around and over the joints are connected to the bones by tendons. When a joint is bent backward or twisted and bent in the abnormal direction, it can cause extreme pain, the ligament can be torn off the bone, and the bones can be pulled apart. Strictly speaking, it is very difficult to use dividing the muscle/tendon and misplacing the bone techniques separately. When one is used, generally the other one is simultaneously applied.

Structure of the joint.

A joint bent backward.

A joint bent and twisted.

## 3. Bi Qi (閉氣) (Sealing the Breath)

"Bi" (閉) in Chinese means "to close, seal, or shut," and "qi" (氣) (more specifically *kong qi*, 空氣) means "air."[4] Bi qi is the technique of preventing the opponent from inhaling, thereby causing him to pass out. There are three categories of bi qi, which differ in their approach to sealing.

Direct sealing by grabbing the throat.

The first category is the direct sealing of the windpipe. You can grab your opponent's throat with your fingers, or compress his throat with your arm, and prevent him from inhaling. Alternatively, you can use your fingers to press or strike the *tiantu* cavity (Co-22, 天突) on the base of his throat to stop him from inhaling. Attacking this area causes the muscles around the windpipe to contract and close the windpipe.

Direct sealing by compressing the throat.

Striking the tiantu cavity.

Tiantu (Co-22)

Tiantu cavity (Co-22).

The second category of bi qi is striking the muscles that surround the lungs. Because of the protection the ribs afford, it is very difficult to strike the muscles around the lungs directly. However, some of these muscles extend beyond the ribs. When they are attacked, they contract in pain and compress the lungs, preventing inhalation. Two muscle groups in the stomach are commonly used in this way.

Rectus abdominis

Striking these stomach muscles can seal the breath.

Finally, the last category of sealing the breath is the cavity press or nerve-ending strike. The principle of this category is very similar to that of the muscle strikes, the only difference being that cavities are struck rather than muscle groups. This category is normally much more difficult, both in principle and technique. However, when it is done correctly, it is more effective than striking the muscles.

If you take a look at the structure of the chest area, you will see that the lungs are well protected by the ribs, which prevent outside forces from damaging the lungs and other organs. You will notice also that each rib is not a single piece of bone wrapping around your body, but rather two pieces of bone, connected by strong ligaments and cartilage. When an outside force strikes the chest, the ribs act like a spring or an elastic ball to bounce the attacking force away or bounce you backward in order to protect the lungs and heart. This construction makes it very hard to cause the lungs to compress by striking the chest. You should also understand that the muscles outside the ribs will not compress the lungs when they contract, because the ribs will protect the lungs. Therefore, in order to cause contraction of the lungs, you must strike particular acupuncture cavities or the ends of the nerves that emerge from the lung area underneath the ribs. Striking these cavities accurately and at the right depth will affect the qi in the muscles around the lungs, causing them to contract. Alternatively, you can strike the nerve endings. This causes pain to penetrate the ribs and shock the internal muscles surrounding the lungs into contraction, thus sealing the breath.

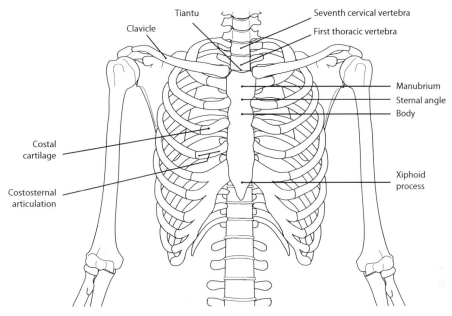

Rib structure of the chest.

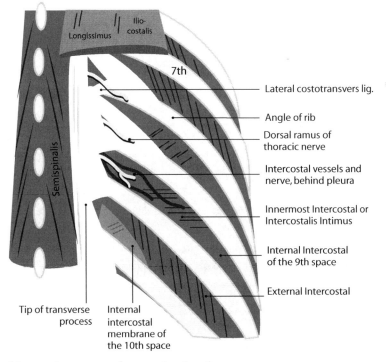

Nerves that emerge from under the ribs.

## 4. Dian Mai or Duan Mai (點脈 / 脈) (Vein/Artery Press or Sealing the Vein/Artery)

"Dian mai" (點脈) is also known as "dim mak," which is simply the same words spoken in a different dialect. "Dian" (點) in Chinese means "to point or press" with a finger. "Mai" means "qi channels" (*qi mai*, 氣脈), or "blood vessels" (*xue mai*, 血脈). Therefore, dian mai means to strike or press either the qi channels or the veins/arteries. When it means to strike or press the vein/artery, it is also called sealing the vein/artery (duan mai). "Duan" (斷) means "to break, seal, or stop." Sometimes it is also called "blood press" (dian xue, 點血), such as when the artery in the temple is struck and ruptured. When dian mai means to strike or press the cavities on the qi channels, it is also called "cavity press" (dian xue, 點穴). Here we will discuss duan mai and leave the discussion of dian xue for later.

In principle, duan mai can be done either by striking or pressing. A striking duan mai qin na can rupture the blood vessel and stop the blood circulation, which usually causes death. For example, when the temple is struck, the muscles in that area will tighten up and rupture the artery. A pressing duan mai qin na can also stop or seal the blood circulation. For example, sealing the neck artery will stop the blood circulation to your head and thus cut down the oxygen supply to the brain. This will cause unconsciousness or even death. There are two major arteries, one on either side of your neck, which supply oxygen to your brain. When either or both of these are struck or pressed, the flow of blood to the brain can be stopped. Sometimes the muscles on the side of the neck remain tensed. CAUTION: These techniques are very dangerous. A person can die from the lack of oxygen that results from sealing the vein/artery. If you do not know how to revive the victim, do not use these techniques.

Striking the taiyang cavity on the temple.

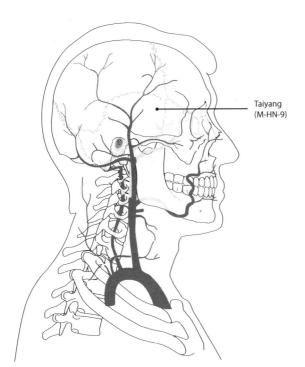

Taiyang
(M-HN-9)

Taiyang cavity on temple.

Pressing the carotid artery on the side of the neck.

Carotid

Artery (carotid) on the side of the neck.

## 5. Dian Mai or Dian Xue (點脈 / 點穴) (Pressing Qi Channel or Pressing Cavity)

As mentioned, the other type of dian mai strikes or presses cavities on qi channels and is also called pressing cavity (dian xue, 點穴). "Dian" (點) means "to press with a finger" and "xue" (穴) refers to the acupuncture cavities. The human body has more than eight hundred qi cavities, mostly on the paths of the eight vessels and twelve channels. Two of the eight vessels are called the governing and conception vessels (*du mai* and *ren mai*, 督脈、任脈). The qi in these two vessels circulates in a twenty-four-hour cycle. The other twelve qi channels are related to the twelve internal organs. The flow of qi in these twelve channels is also related to the time of the day, with emphasis switching from one channel to the next gradually, every two hours. Furthermore, these eight vessels and twelve channels also have seasonal and annual cycles. When the qi circulation in these vessels and channels is stagnant or stopped, the person will sicken or die. Acupuncture is a way to readjust the qi circulation and cure illness.

Cavity press is a method to disturb or affect the opponent's qi circulation. There are about 108 cavities that can be struck or pressed to affect the qi flow. Among these 108 cavities, strikes to thirty-six can cause death, and strikes to the other seventy-two can cause numbness or unconsciousness. In order to make a strike effective, you must know the time of the major qi flow (*zi wu liu zhu*, 子午流注) in that channel, the appropriate striking technique, and the depth of the cavity. We will not go into greater detail in this book, both because it is a very complicated subject, and because it can be very dangerous for a person to learn without supervision. In traditional Chinese martial society, a master will usually not pass these secrets on until he feels he can really trust a student. However, some techniques can be taught without too much danger. These cavities will not cause death, and most are attacked through the method called grabbing the cavity (*zhua xue*, 抓穴). If you are interested in some information about qi flow and its timing, please refer to *Qigong for Health and Martial Arts*, published by YMAA.

Often when cavities are pressed, it is accomplished by both striking and pressing. When pressing is used, normally it gets involved in the grabbing. Therefore, some Chinese martial artists again divide cavity attacks into cavity striking (*da xue*, 打穴) and cavity grabbing or pressing (*na xue* or *dian xue*, 拿穴、點穴). Cavity striking is classified in the category of striking, while cavity grabbing or pressing belongs to the category of qin na.

There is another category that may make you confused. Often, the nerves near the joint areas are grabbed to numb or to immobilize joint movements. However, the areas in which the nerves are commonly exposed for grabbing are also in the same locations as the cavities. In other words, the cavities and the nerve grabbing are in the same spot.

Because of this, it is misrepresented that this kind of grabbing is cavity pressing or nerve grabbing. Strictly speaking, this kind of grabbing should be classified as cavity pressing.

Before we finish this section, you should understand that in Chinese martial arts you must have jing to make your techniques effective. Jing is a way of expressing power that makes the power stronger and more penetrating. When jing is expressed, the muscles and tendons are supported by the qi in the body, so that the muscles and tendons reach their highest efficiency. Jing can be categorized as hard, soft-hard, or soft. When you apply a qin na, regardless of which category it falls into, if you do not know how to use your jing in the technique, your qin na will be ineffective. For example, if you do not use jing in "dividing the muscle/tendon" (fen jin) qin na, your opponent will have an opportunity to use his muscles to resist your muscles. If you do not use a jerking jing in "misplacing the bone" (cuo gu) qin na, you will not be able to break or misplace the opponent's joint. In the same way, in a sealing-the-breath or cavity-press technique, if no jing is used, the power will not penetrate to the right depth and the technique will be ineffective. For a greater understanding of jing, refer to the author's book *Tai Chi Theory and Martial Power, published by YMAA.*

## 1-3. Different Levels of Qin Na Techniques

As with most Chinese martial arts, qin na is composed of many different levels, according to different criteria or standards. In this section we would like to define these standards according to several different systems of categorization.

First, the levels of qin na techniques can be divided according to how much a person understands the technique and the technical difficulty of the technique executed. The same techniques—based on the same theory and principle—can generate very different results, according to an individual's expertise. Normally, this can be judged according to a few common criteria. First, a beginner's power is usually dull and stagnant, and therefore the technique is executed slowly and poorly. When an expert is performing the same technique, his power is soft and gentle, and therefore his technique is fast and effective. Second, a beginner usually cannot catch the correct angle of locking through the feel of the contact, while an expert can grasp the correct angle instinctively. Generally, this instinct will take many months of diligent practice for each technique until they become natural and smooth. This is also the reason a beginner needs to use more muscular, slow power.

Third, when a technique is applied by a beginner, the victim can feel the angle as it occurs, but when done by a qin na expert, the victim will feel nothing until he is locked in place. The reason for this is that an expert will use a flowing, circular motion. When this circular motion is used, usually you will not realize you are being locked, and therefore your reaction will not be as instinctive and automatic as when someone tries to lock you at an obvious angle. Finally, when a beginner is executing a technique, usually he does not know how to coordinate his breathing and mind, and therefore the technique is not executed as effectively as it would be by an expert. This is like when you use an ax to chop a piece of wood. If you know how to place your mind on the bottom of the wood you would like to chop and how to coordinate with your exhalation, you will find you can break the wood much more easily than you could without such concentration.

Next, the levels of qin na techniques can be very different according to different martial styles. For example, "small wrap hand" wrist qin na is one of the most common techniques based on the theory of dividing the muscle/tendon. However, because of different understanding and training methods in various martial styles, it can be used to accomplish distinctly different results, and its effectiveness can also vary. Although ostensibly the same technique, some martial styles will execute it with good speed and an accurate locking angle, while others go slowly and remain on the surface. This means that even the same technique can vary in its effectiveness, depending on the styles, the teacher, and the student.

Next, the levels of qin na techniques can be distinguished according to different qin na categories discussed in the previous sections. Generally speaking, the theory and the techniques of the "dividing muscle/tendon" and "misplacing the bone" qin na techniques are the easiest to learn and apply. "Grabbing the tendon" qin na is harder since it needs more strength, accuracy, and concentration to make it work. In some advanced "grabbing tendon" qin na, the qi and the coordination of the breathing are required. "Sealing the vein/artery" are the third most difficult techniques to learn. Although some of the "sealing the vein/artery" qin na techniques applied to the neck are fairly easy to learn, most of the others are much more difficult and require special training. Finally, "pressing cavity" qin na is the hardest since it requires in-depth knowledge about the locations of cavities, the application of specific hand forms and techniques, the time window of vulnerability associated with each cavity, and the depth of penetration required for your power to properly affect the cavity. According to Chinese medicine, qi circulates in the body's qi channels and is affected and significantly influenced by the time of day and the seasons of the year. Furthermore, in order to effectively use even a small number of "pressing cavity" techniques, jing training is required. Normally, it will take a person more than ten years of vigorous practice to understand these theories and reach the final mastery of "pressing cavity" qin na.

Remember, a good qin na is not necessarily complicated. Soon, you will realize that the simple techniques are usually faster and easier to apply. Very often, this helps make them more effective than those techniques that look fancy but take a lot of time to apply. The key to judging a good technique is to decide how fast and effective the technique is when it is applied. Also, you should remember that almost all of the qin na techniques are related to the mutual angle between you and your opponent. When you set up an angle for locking, if your opponent is experienced, he can sense it and remove the angle. Furthermore, he may mount a counter qin na technique to lock you. Therefore, the longer the time you take when you execute a technique, the greater the chance your opponent will be able to escape or even counterattack. When two qin na experts are practicing qin na, it is continuous, without an end. The reason for this is simply because every qin na can be countered, and every countered qin na can be countered. Therefore, if both practitioners are able to feel or sense the attacks clearly and accurately, either one will be able to change the locking angle to free himself and immediately execute another qin na on his opponent. Naturally, to reach this stage, you will need many years of practice and accumulation of experience.

Finally, you should understand that in order to reach an in-depth level of qin na, you should follow the training procedures that have been used in the past. First, you should regulate your body until all of the physical positions are accurate. This includes the mutual angle for locking, the positioning of your body, and the correct posture for controlling. After you have mastered all of these factors, you should then regulate your breathing. Correct breathing helps to manifest your power to a stronger stage. You will also need to regulate your mind. Remember, your mind leads the qi (or bioelectricity) to the muscles and tendons to activate them for action. The more your mind can be concentrated, the more qi can be led, and the more power you can generate. It is said, "Yi arrives, qi also arrives" ("Yi dao, qi yi dao").[5] Once you have regulated your body, breathing, mind, and qi, then you can raise up your spirit of controlling. This will lead you to the final level of perfect technique execution. If you are interested in knowing more about this external and internal training, please refer to *The Root of Chinese Qigong*, published by YMAA.

## 1-4. Qin Na and Health

If a person has never practiced qin na before, the painful feeling that comes through practice may cause him to jump to the conclusion that qin na is only for martial arts. In fact, only those people who have practiced qin na for some time realize that through practicing qin na, they can gain many health benefits, both physical and mental. In this section, let us address some of the health benefits we are able to gain from practicing qin na.

### Mental Health

1. **Increase awareness.** The first benefit a qin na practitioner gains is building the sense of awareness. This begins with an awareness of the angles that can be harmful to the joints, tendons, and muscles. Qin na specializes in locking the joints through the angles you set up, especially the angles affecting the tendons and ligaments. Through training, a practitioner learns to be aware of the angles that can be harmful

to the body. Naturally, he will also build up an awareness of how to avoid the angles that can cause injury to the joints. You should remember that most bodily injury is to the joints and is caused by using adverse angles of force or postures.

2. **Build up the mental endurance and establish a strong will.** After only five minutes of practice, every qin na beginner will realize that practicing qin na is a painful process. This pain is not only from the physical twisting and locking of the joints. It is also from mental struggling. We should understand that our life is painful and that our minds are always in conflict. According to Chinese philosophy and understanding, a human has two minds: the emotional mind (*xin*, 心) and the wisdom mind (*yi*, 意). These two minds often conflict with each other. On one hand, the wisdom mind knows what we should or shouldn't do. But on the other hand, the emotional mind makes a person always end up on the path to sensory satisfaction. Everybody knows that the wisdom mind is clear and has wise judgment. Unfortunately, we often surrender to our emotional mind and suppress our wisdom mind.

One of the main purposes of training Chinese martial arts is to establish a discipline that trains you how to use your wisdom mind to govern your emotional mind. Only then will you have a strong will. Both physical and mental hardships are necessary to accomplish this goal. When you practice qin na, you know both that it will be painful and that you must build up your endurance to deal with this pain in order to learn. As a matter of fact, learning qin na is just like any other traditional martial art—a method of self-challenge. Through this challenge, you will be able to understand yourself better and be more capable of comprehending the meaning of your life.

3. **Understand the human qi body.** In order to control your opponents effectively, along with understanding the structure of the human physical body, you should also understand the human qi body. For example, in order to make cavity press qin na effective (cavity press uses grabbing, striking, or finger pressing to affect the body's qi circulation), you must have a good understanding of the distribution of qi in your opponent's body and the correct depth and timing of your attack.

According to Chinese medicine and qigong practice, a person has two bodies, the physical body and the qi body. Western medicine has reached a very high level in understanding the physical body. However, its understanding of the qi body is still in its infancy. If you are able to understand both your physical body and your qi body, you will be able to regulate your bodies to a healthier state. If you are interested in understanding more about the qi body, please refer to the book *The Root of Chinese Qigong*, published by YMAA.

4. **Train mental balance, stability, center, and root.** According to Chinese medicine and martial arts, in order to have good physical balance, stability, and centering, you

must first have mental balance, stability, and centering. You should understand that the mind is the master that governs and controls the actions of your physical body. If your mind is confused and scattered, this will not only affect your decisions, but will also destroy the feeling of your physical balance and center. In addition, when you have firm mental balance, stability, centering, and rooting, you will also be able to build up your spirit of vitality.

One qin na training consists of "takedown" techniques. In this category of training, you learn how to firm your center and root while at the same time finding your opponent's center and root to destroy them. By understanding the relationship between your own mental state and root, you will better be able to attack your enemy's spirit and consequently disrupt his physical coordination.

5. **Make friends.** One of the invisible benefits of qin na training, like all other sports, is that through practice you can make so many friends. I am amazed at how often I rediscover this benefit. I have traveled to more than twelve countries in the last eight years, and have made thousands of friends. This has filled my life with more love and meaning.

## Physical Health

1. **Stretching the physical body.** Two of the qin na categories are "misplacing the bone" and "dividing the muscle/tendon." These two categories specialize in locking the joints through twisting and bending. Unless you are using qin na against an enemy, when you practice with your partner you will usually not twist and bend the ligaments or tendons beyond their limit, which can cause injury. Because of this, qin na training has become one the best ways to stretch the joints.

According to Chinese medicine and qigong, the more we stimulate our physical body properly, the more the blood and qi circulation can be improved. A healthy condition can be improved and strength and endurance can be increased. In fact, this is the basic theory behind yoga. Through twisting and stretching, the deep places in the joints can be stimulated and strength can be maintained. Like yoga, from countless practitioners' experience, qin na has been proven one of the best methods of stretching the joints.

2. **Understanding the structure of the physical body.** In order to make qin na effective, you must also know the structure of the joints and how the muscles and tendons relate to the action or movement of the body. Through practicing qin na, you will be able to gain a clearer picture of this structure. Only through understanding this physical structure may you reduce or prevent physical damage or injury to your body.

3. **Learning how to heal yourself.** Truly speaking, no matter how carefully both you and your partner pay attention, you will eventually experience some sort of minor injury during the learning process. The reasons for this are, first, you and your partner are excited during learning and are expecting some painful reaction from each other. Understanding this condition, you both may use power that is beyond the limits you can endure. Second, since both you and your partner are beginners, you do not yet have enough experience to see how much power you should apply to each other. This can result in injury. Normally, injury does not occur with experienced practitioners.

Once you have an injury, you will learn how to move it correctly, how to massage it, how to relax it, and how to apply herbs to expedite the healing process.

4. **Firming physical balance, stability, centering, and root.** We have discussed earlier the importance of mental and physical balance, stability, centering, and root, and how they relate to each other. Here I would like to remind you that through practicing qin na, you will be able to coordinate your mental and physical centers smoothly and comfortably.

## 1-5. Differences between Shaolin Qin Na and Taiji Qin Na

Strictly speaking, it is very hard to distinguish the differences in qin na as applied from within external martial styles and internal martial styles. The reason for this is simply because no matter how or from what the qin na is created and applied, it is all based on the same theories of locking (dividing the muscle/tendon and misplacing the bone), sealing (sealing the vein or artery), and pressing (striking or pressing the cavities). In addition, no matter which style a martial artist has practiced, when he has reached a high level of qin na expertise, he should be so skillful that all techniques can be executed softly and circularly.

This is similar to the differences between external martial styles and internal martial styles. Many people think that the techniques in the external styles are hard and that only muscular power is used to execute the techniques. They also believe that external stylists do not train the cultivation of qi. In fact, this is not true. In Chinese martial society, it is said, "External styles from external to internal, and internal styles from internal to external; though the path is opposite, the final goal is the same."[6] This means that external martial artists start with the external, training to use muscular power to execute their techniques first. Then gradually they will minimize the usage of the muscles and train to cultivate the internal qi to energize the muscles to their maximum usage. This is exactly the opposite approach from the internal stylists, who start with the cultivation of qi first and gradually apply the qi to the muscles to execute their techniques. There is a well-known proverb that says: "Externally train tendons, bones, and skin; internally train a mouthful of qi."[7] This means a martial artist should learn how to train the physical body to be strong, and he should also train internal qi. The proverb refers to the mouthful of qi because breathing is closely related to the cultivation of qi.

From this you can see that when a martial artist reaches a high level of training, it does not matter if he is an internal or external stylist: The final goal of training is the same. However, if we take a detailed look at the differences in the external styles' qin na and the internal styles' qin na, we can reach several general conclusions.

1. Shaolin Qin Na is a harder style, while taiji qin na is a softer style. Because there are different training methods for the beginner in taiji versus Shaolin, generally speaking the applications of Shaolin Qin Na are harder, while taiji qin na are softer. This implies that Shaolin Qin Na uses more muscles, while taiji qin na uses more qi.

2. Shaolin Qin Na emphasizes both straight and round movements, while taiji qin na movements are usually rounder. This distinction is again a result of the differences between the basic training principles. Shaolin emphasizes both straight and round actions; taiji principles focus mainly on round movements.

3. Relatively speaking, Shaolin Qin Na is more offensive and aggressive, while taiji qin na is more defensive and passive. The strategy of Shaolin martial arts emphasizes both defense and offense, while taiji specializes in using defense as offense. Relatively speaking, Shaolin Qin Na is more offensive, while taiji qin na is more defensive.

Even though we have examined the differences between Shaolin and taiji qin na, you should not be restricted by these differences. A good martial artist and qin na expert should master both hard and soft techniques. This means that when it is necessary to be soft, you are able to be soft, and when it is necessary to be hard, you can be hard. Only then can you say you are a qin na expert.

## 1-6. About This Book

Before continuing to read this book, you should understand a few important points:

1. This book can only offer you some qin na techniques with which I am familiar. To tell the truth, many of these qin na techniques originated from my White Crane and Long Fist background. The reason for this is simply that the martial applications of taijiquan have been ignored in the last fifty years. Many of the martial techniques have been lost. Qin na is one of the typical examples. Even though taijiquan greatly emphasizes qin na, it is nearly impossible to find a master, even in China today, who is an expert in it. Naturally, there is no book available. Fortunately, since

qin na theory and its basic principles of application remain the same, this allows me to trace back some of the possible qin na applications in taijiquan. I hope from the publication of this book that sincere study and research of this subject can be conducted. If you are interested in knowing more about the martial applications of taijiquan, you may read the book *Tai Chi Chuan Martial Applications*, published by YMAA.

2. Behind every joint-locking qin na technique, there is always one or more hidden striking techniques that can be used to injure or kill your opponent. This was necessary, especially in ancient times, when guns were not available. Often in battle, due to slippage from sweat or the exceptional strength of an opponent, joint-locking qin na becomes ineffective. When this happens, you will be forced to injure or kill your opponent instead of mercifully controlling him. In fact, qin na techniques often served only for temporarily locking the opponent, which can therefore create a safe opportunity for your further attacking or taking down.

3. In the same fighting situation, there can be many possible qin na techniques and options. Some techniques may be more effective and powerful for some opponents, while others may be easier to apply for some other opponents. Some techniques emphasize speed more than strength, while others may rely on physical strength. The most important point is that you should treat all of the techniques as alive, and adapt them wisely and skillfully depending on the situation. This means that when you apply your techniques, you must consider your size, power, height, and skill.

4. If you apply them skillfully and circularly, techniques from other styles can be adapted and be made soft. When they are soft and round, it will be harder for your opponent to sense his danger. Actually, in the higher levels of qin na, techniques can be applied so softly that muscular usage is reduced to a minimum. Naturally, the thought of execution is stronger and more focused, and this enables the qi to circulate smoothly and abundantly to energize the muscles to a state of higher efficiency.

5. In order to effectively control your opponent and immediately put him into an awkward and submissive situation, jerking martial power (*fa jing*, 發勁) is often necessary. Once you have locked your opponent into an accurate angle, if you apply jerking martial power, you may immediately lock or injure him efficiently. Naturally, if you practice with your friends, you should not do this, since it can detach the ligaments from the bones, tear off the tendons, disconnect the joints, or even break the bones. If you are interested in knowing more about martial power (jing), you may refer to the book *Tai Chi Theory and Martial Power*, published by YMAA.

6. Though some cavity press qin na are also included in this book, these techniques only serve as a reference. From the discussion of these techniques, you may obtain some idea of how and why cavity press qin na works. Cavity press techniques are

considered one of the highest skills in Chinese martial arts. Naturally, it will take you many years of learning and practice under a proficient master to reach this high level. To discuss this subject in a few pages is not possible. In fact, it is very difficult to write about this subject clearly in book form since a great deal of information about training and applications is from the master's experience.

7. In every qin na technique, there is always one or more counter technique. Again, in every one of these counter techniques, there is also one or more counter-counter techniques. That means that if your qin na techniques are very skillful and you are able to achieve the right timing, you will be able to counter any qin na. Since most of the counterattack qin na have been discussed in the book *Analysis of Shaolin Chin Na*, published by YMAA, we will not repeat them here.

In order to have a better foundation, in addition to reading this book, you should also read *Analysis of Shaolin Chin Na*. This book will help you build up a firm theoretical foundation and classify all of the different techniques. In addition, if you are interested in knowing how qin na is applied in an actual combat situation, you may refer to the book *Comprehensive Applications of Shaolin Chin Na*, published by YMAA.

Although this book can offer you theory and pictures, it cannot offer you the continuous movement of the action. With the help of the companion video, you will be able to see the action, and this will lead you to a better understanding of how a technique can be executed. Finally, even if you have books and video, if you do not have the correct feeling, you will often miss the key angles and points for effective locking. Participating in qin na seminars offered by qualified masters is also highly recommended. From seminars, you can be led onto the right path in just a few days or even a few hours. This could save you a lot of confusion and wondering.

Next, you should always have a humble and appreciative mind. Those who are humble and appreciative will continue to absorb knowledge, while those who become satisfied will become impervious to it. It is said in Chinese society, "Satisfaction loses and humility gains."[8]

In the second chapter, basic taiji technical moving patterns and their martial application theories will be discussed. Only after you have understood these basic moving patterns will you be able to understand how they can be used in qin na and how qin na can be used against these moving patterns. In the third and fourth chapters, qin na techniques that can be used both from and against these patterns will be introduced. Then, in the fifth chapter, we will summarize those qin na techniques that can be used in thirty-seven Yang Style Taijiquan postures. Finally, in the sixth chapter, in order to help you understand how taiji qin na can be applied in taiji pushing hands situations, some examples will be highlighted.

Finally, Chinese masters always say: "Practice makes perfect." You should practice, practice, and then practice. The only trick to perfecting an art once you understand the basic theories and principles is constant practice. From practice, your techniques will become ever more skillful, and your understanding will grow ever deeper. Remember, when you practice with a partner, you should avoid hurting each other intentionally. Always control your power. A good martial artist should always know how to control his power. Some qin na injuries can be permanent. For example, once a ligament is detached from the bones in the joint, the damage will be permanent, and the only way to repair it is through surgery.

## References

1. Throwing down qin na is often also classified as a part of the Chinese wrestling (shuai jiao).
2. "Mai" here means "xue mai" and translates to "blood vessels."
3. "Mai" here means "qi mai" and translates to "primary qi channels."
4. The word "qi" in Chinese can mean two things, depending on its context. The first meaning is air (kong qi), and the second is the energy that circulates in the human body. Unless otherwise noted, "qi" in this book denotes this second meaning.
5. 意到，氣亦到。
6. 外家由外而內，內家由內而外，其途雖異，其終的卻一致。
7. 外練筋骨皮，內練一口氣。
8. 滿招損，謙受益。

# Chapter 2: Basic Taiji Theory

## 2-1. Introduction

If we desire to understand taiji theory, then we must first trace back to its origins and roots. Only then will we know how and where it came from. Although a great proportion of Chinese martial arts history is vague, we can still trace it with some accuracy and in some detail.

If we trace Chinese martial arts history back, we can see a clear lineage beginning during the Liang dynasty (梁朝) (AD 502–557). There are no surviving martial documents from before this time that record or discuss qi and how to correlate it with martial arts, even though at that time, Chinese qigong practice had existed for more than two thousand years. It is understood that before the Chinese Han dynasty (漢朝) (206 BC–AD 221), there were only two schools of qigong practice: the medical group and the scholarly group. It was not until the East Han dynasty (東漢) (circa AD 58) that Buddhist qigong was imported to China from India. Still, even then very little training theory and methods were passed down. The many Buddhist holy writings or Chinese classics a student could obtain were purely the doctrines of Buddhism and talked very little about how to cultivate qi internally.

This situation lasted until the Chinese Liang dynasty, when Da Mo (達摩) was invited to China to preach in front of the emperor. However, because Emperor Liang Wu (梁武帝) did not favor Da Mo's Buddhist theories and means of cultivation, Da Mo was forced to retire to the Shaolin Temple. Before Da Mo died in the temple, he passed down two classics on the cultivation of qi, the *Yi Jin Jing* and the *Xi Sui Jing* (易筋經, 洗髓經), which can help a practitioner to enter a state of enlightenment or Buddhahood.

From Da Mo's classics, the Shaolin monks trained the cultivation of qi and realized that from this cultivation, muscular power could be enhanced to a tremendous level, which could make martial techniques more powerful and effective. This was the beginning of internal cultivation in the martial arts. According to ancient records, it was only about fifty years later that internal styles based on Da Mo's internal qi cultivation were created. Two of the best known of these styles are small nine heaven (*xiao jiu tian*, 小九天) and post-heaven techniques (*hou tian fa*, 後天法).[1] All of these styles were created based on the same taiji theories and principles known today. These theories and principles are as follows:

1. Qi should be first cultivated and developed internally, then this qi is slowly manifested as power through the physical body, and finally it is applied into the techniques.

2. In order to allow the qi to circulate smoothly and freely in the body, the physical body must first be relaxed, and the movements must be soft.

3. The *yin* and *yang* theory and concepts are the foundations and root of qi development. From this we can see that the roots of taijiquan have existed for at least thirteen hundred years. Within this time, thousands of techniques have been discovered and hundreds of styles have been created. Moreover, the very theoretical underpinnings of taijiquan have been studied and researched continuously. From the accumulation of thought, its theories have reached a very profound level, even as its contents have expanded into an ever-wider range.

The implication of this is that these two styles were probably the progenitors of taijiquan. It is believed that taijiquan was not actually named "taijiquan" until the Chinese Song dynasty (宋朝) (circa AD 1101). Chang, San-feng (張三豐) is widely credited as the creator of taijiquan.

From surviving fragments of documents from this time, it can be surmised that the Shaolin Temple was the major influence on the development of qi cultivation in martial arts society. It is therefore valid to imply that substantial taijiquan theory originated at the temple. In fact, if we look to contemporary Chen Style Taijiquan, similarities emerge between it and certain external Shaolin styles. For example, both the first and second routines—*changquan* (長拳) and cannon fist (*pao chui*, 炮捶)—originated at the Shaolin Temple, yet they also exist in Chen Style (even the names were kept the same as those in the temple). Although the Shaolin changquan and pao chui have been modified and revised in Chen Style Taijiquan, we can still trace back the root and origin of every movement clearly in today's Chen Style Taijiquan. This holds true for many of the taijiquan weapons routines.

It is well known that Yang Style originated from Chen Style and that they still share the same taiji root and essence. Wu and Sun Styles originated from Yang Style. From this we can see that taijiquan and Shaolin martial arts in fact share the same root. It is no wonder that many taijiquan masters who have also learned Shaolin martial arts are more expert and proficient in the martial roots and applications of taijiquan. The reason for this is simply because the "Dao" of Chinese martial arts remains the same in all Chinese styles. Different styles are only different variations and derivations (branches and flowers) from the same root. When you learn different styles, you will have different angles from which to view the same "Dao" (道). Naturally, your mind can be clearer, and your understanding can be more profound.

Now, let us see what "taijiquan" is, as written down in the past. First, we must define what we mean by "taiji." It is said,

> What is taiji? It is generated from wuji. It is the mother of yin and yang. When it moves, it divides. At rest it reunites. [1, 2]
>
> 太極者，無極而生，陰陽之母也，動之則分，靜之則合。

Taiji can be translated as "grand ultimate" or "grand extremity." That refers to the most essential movements, or the very origin of motivation or force. *Wuji* (無極) means "no extremity," and means "no dividing" or "no discrimination." Wuji is a state of formlessness, of staying in the center: calm, quiet, and peaceful. When you are in the wuji state, there is no form or shape. Once you have generated a mind or have formed the mental shape with which you will influence physical reality, the motivation of dividing or discriminating starts. When this dividing is happening, wuji will become yin and yang. From this you can see what taiji is: it is the motivation of distinguishment. When you have this motivation, the qi will then be led, and yin and yang can be distinguished.

Once this motivation (taiji) stops, the motivator of division stops, and the yin and yang will once again reunite and return to wuji. From this you can see that taiji is actually the motive force generated from the mind (yi, 意). From this force, the qi is led and circulates throughout the body. We can therefore conclude that taijiquan is the martial style that trains the practitioner to use the mind to lead the qi, circulating it in the body and consequently generating the yin and yang states for health, fighting, or improving longevity.

Again, taijiquan is also called long fist (changquan, 長拳). It is said,

> What is long fist? [It is] like a long river and a large ocean, rolling ceaselessly. [1]
>
> 長拳者，如長江大海滔滔不絕也。

Originally, the name "changquan" came from the Shaolin Temple. "Changquan" means "long fist." It can also be translated as "long range" or "long sequence." Ancient documents suggest that the meaning of "changquan" in taijiquan means the "long sequence," like a long river that acts as a conduit to the open ocean. The qi circulating in the body is rolling continuously, flowing and ebbing in natural cycles.

Taijiquan is also called thirteen postures (*shi san shi*, 十三勢). It is said,

> What are the thirteen postures? Peng, lu, ji, an, cai, lie, zhou, kou; these are the eight trigrams. Jin bu, tui bu, zuo gu, you pan, zhong ding; these are the five elements. Peng, lu, ji, an are qian [heaven], kun [earth], kan [water], li [fire]; these are the four main sides. Cai, lie, zhou, kou are xun [wind], zhen [thunder], dui

[lake], and gen [mountain]: the four diagonal corners. Jin bu, tui bu, zuo gu, you pan, and zhong ding are jin [metal] mu [wood], shui [water], huo [fire], and tu [earth]. All together they are the thirteen postures.[1]

十三勢者，掤、搌、擠、按、採、捌、肘、靠，此八卦也。進步、退步、左顧、右盼、中定，此五行也。掤、搌、擠、按，即乾、坤、坎、離，四正方也。採、捌、肘、靠，即巽、震、兌、艮，四斜角也。進、退、顧、盼、定，即金、木、水、火、土也。合之為十三勢也。

Taijiquan includes eight basic moving or martial power (jing, 勁) patterns, which are considered the eight corners of the eight trigrams. *Peng* (掤), *lu* (搌), *ji* (擠), and *an* (按) are considered the four sides of the eight trigrams, while *cai* (採), *lie* (捌), *zhou* (肘), and *kao* (靠) are regarded as the four diagonal corners. Taijiquan also contains five basic strategic movements or steppings: forward (*jin bu*, 進步), backward (*tui bu*, 退步), see the left (*zuo gu*, 左顧), look to the right (*you pan*, 右盼), and firm the center (*zhong ding*, 中定).

From this you can see that these thirteen postures are actually the foundation of taijiquan. From these thirteen postures, hundreds of techniques and strategic movements can be generated. As in a waltz, though there are only three steps in the basic movement, the variations can number in the hundreds. Therefore, in order to understand the qin na applications of taijiquan, you must first become familiar with the qin na hidden in these thirteen postures, and you must also know the qin na that can be used against these thirteen postures.

Taijiquan has also been called san shi qi shi (三十七勢), which means "thirty-seven postures." The reason for this is that if you count the technique movements or postures of Yang Style Taijiquan, you will find that they number only thirty-seven. However, it is from these thirty-seven postures that more than 250 martial applications are derived. Naturally, these thirty-seven postures are also built upon the foundation of the "thirteen postures" or "thirteen jing patterns and strategies." In fact, many of these thirty-seven postures are constructed from two or more of the original thirteen jing patterns. For example, wave hands in clouds and grasp sparrow's tail are the combinations of peng jing and lie jing. From this you can see that the original thirteen patterns first evolve into thirty-seven basic postures or movements, and that these thirty-seven basic postures can themselves be divided into hundreds of techniques and variations.

## 2-2. The Three Different Fighting Ranges and Circles

Within Chinese martial arts, fighting ranges also differ according to style and strategy. Generally, fighting ranges can be divided into three categories: long (長), medium (中), and short (短). In the long range, the distance between you and your opponent is beyond the reach of your legs; you cannot reach each other without stepping forward. Normally, this is the safest range, since neither of you are at a distance from which any move-

ment can be made without the other having a chance to react.

In the medium range, the distance between you and your opponent is closer. In this range either of you can reach the other with a kick. Naturally, this is more dangerous for both sides; when you enter this range, you must be very alert. Whoever attacks first may have the advantage of tim-

Long-range fighting distance.

ing and can put his opponent into a defensive situation. Often this range is used to execute a faking technique first, setting up further attacks or creating an opportunity to move into the short range.

Medium-range fighting distance.

Short-range fighting distance.

Finally, in the short range, the distance between you and your opponent is so close that either of you can reach the other simply by extending an arm. When you and your opponent are at such a short distance, both of you must be extremely alert, since either one of you can attack the other with great speed and surprise.

Therefore, when you fight, you want to keep the distance between you and your opponent in the long range. Only when you have an opportunity should you enter the medium or short ranges. Once you are in the medium and short ranges, you must react immediately to any change. This strategy is the same in taijiquan fighting. However, since taijiquan strategy uses defense as offense, you usually must wait for your opponent's attack. Once your opponent attacks you, use your hands to intercept and stick to the attack. Then you can shorten the distance between you and your opponent from the long range into the medium and short ranges, and at the same time you can adhere your hands to his arms or body. From taiji pushing hands training, you learn how to stick and adhere and practice how to destroy your opponent's balance. Once your opponent loses his balance and his mind focuses on regaining it, immediately separate the adhering hands and attack. From this you can see that taijiquan fighting strategy and methods are different from most external styles, in which sticking and adhering are not the main training objectives.

After you know the three ranges, then you should learn about the three circles in taijiquan: large (大), medium (中), and small (小) circles. When you initially intercept your opponent's attack, your arms are widely extended. If you fight in this long extended arm circle, it is called "large circle" (*da quan*, 大圈). In this circle, realistically speaking, it is very hard to keep your hands adhered to your opponent's arm. However, if you immediately close into the medium circle (*zhong quan*, 中圈), in which your arms are half bent, then the adhering maneuvers become much easier and more practical. This is simply because your arms have more extending and shortening range in which to move for the purpose of adhering at this distance. In this circle, you have to compete with your opponent to see who is more capable of destroying the other's balance, thus creating an opportunity for attack.

When a proficient taiji expert has reached a very high level of fighting skill, then he will gradually learn how to close still more and fight in the small circle (*xiao quan*, 小圈). Since your skills are much higher than those of your opponent in this circle, you are able to attack in such a short range without fail. The reason is that in such a short range, the attack can be so fast that it is almost impossible to react to the attack successfully. This is why it is said, "The higher the skills are, the smaller the circle will be."[3]

Large circle.

Medium circle.

Now that you understand the differences in the three ranges and the three circles, in the next section we would like to discuss the eight most important taiji moving patterns and the five strategic movements—together called the thirteen postures.

Small circle.

## 2-3. The Thirteen Postures

In this section, we will define the eight basic taiji technical moving patterns: peng, lu, ji, *an*, cai, lie, zhou, and kao, and the five important taiji strategic directional movements: forward, backward, left, right, and center, which comprise the thirteen postures. Since these eight technical patterns and five strategic movements are the main body of taijiquan, before we discuss the qin na applications of taijiquan, you should first clearly understand the meaning of these thirteen postures.

### I. Eight Basic Technical Moving Patterns

### 1. Peng (掤)

Peng can be translated as "wardoff." Peng has the feeling of roundness and expansion. Generally, this round and expanding feeling is formed and generated from the chest and the arm(s). For example, when you use your arm to push people away with the support of the arcing chest, it is called *peng kai* (掤開), which means "open with wardoff." The expanding force can be upward, forward, or sideways.

Peng force. Opening with wardoff (peng kai).

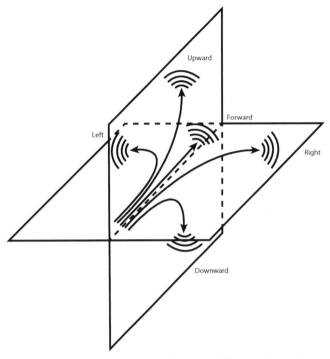

Peng kai force can be expressed upward, forward, or sideways.

The force generated from peng is very offensive and forceful, just like a beach ball bouncing you away. Peng is often used to generate a circular defensive force by the chest and the arms. This allows you a chance to apply wardoff against the opponent's power, redirecting it upward and thereby neutralizing his attacking force.

Peng force. Upward.

The typical examples of peng force in taijiquan postures are wardoff (forward or slightly upward), grasp sparrow's tail (upward), wave hands in clouds (sideways), and crane spreads its wings (upward diagonally).

Peng (wardoff) applied. Begins with forward force then moves slightly upward.

Peng (wardoff) applied. Grasp sparrow's tail uses upward peng force.

Peng applied. Wave hands in clouds uses sideways peng force.

Peng applied. Crane spreads its wings uses upward diagonal peng force.

## 2. Lu (擺)

Lu means "to yield, lead, and neutralize"; it is commonly translated as "rollback." The main purpose of this movement is to yield the force first, then to lead it backward and to the side for neutralizing. Theoretically, lu is a defensive strategic movement. However, occasionally, lu can be aggressive when the timing and situation allow. For example, when you yield and lead, you may also lock or break the opponent's arm.

Lu force. Yield, lead, and neutralize.

Lu force is aggressive.

In Chinese martial arts, lu can be applied in two ways. One is to first apply wardoff against the opponent's arm with your arm, and then to rollback his arm, backward and to your side. This rollback action is also called small rollback (*xiao lu*, 小擺).

Lu applied. Begin by using wardoff (external intercept).

Using small rollback to finish the technique.

Lu applied. Begin by using wardoff (internal intercept).

Using small rollback to finish the technique.

The other case is to use one of your hands to grab your opponent's wrist while using the forearm of the other arm to press and lock the rear side of his post-arm (upper arm). This kind of rollback is called large rollback (*da lu*, 大擺).

Lu applied. Using large rollback to finish the technique.

## 3. Ji (擠)

Ji is defined as "squeeze" or "press." This action can be performed with two hands, where the palms face and then press against each other. Alternatively, the ji force can also be performed by pressing forward with both hands, forearms, or one hand to the other arm.

Ji force. Press or squeeze.

Ji applied. Pressing forward with both hands.

Ji applied. Pressing forward with the forearm.

Ji applied. Pressing forward with one hand on the other arm.

## 4. An (按)

*An* means "stamp" or "press down, forward, or upward." *An* can be done with both hands or with a single hand. *An* action is generally performed with the fingers pointing forward first and then, right before reaching the target, the wrist is angled downward, forward, or upward. This kind of action is called "settling the wrist."

*An* force. Using two hands.

*An* force. Using one hand.

*An* force begins with fingers pointing forward.

Then settle the wrist downward.

Alternative: Settle the wrist forward.

Alternative: Settle the wrist upward.

*An* is commonly used to seal the opponent's arm or joints, or for attacking his abdominal area by pressing downward. It is also often used to attack the opponent's chest by pressing forward or pressing upward.

*An* applied. Sealing the opponent's arm or joints.

*An* applied. Pressing downward on the abdomen.

*An* applied. Pressing forward on the chest.

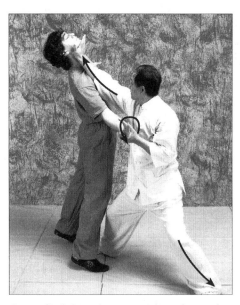

*An* applied. Pressing upward on the neck.

## 5. Cai (採)

Cai stands for "pluck" or "grab." This is the action of locking the opponent's joints, such as the elbow or wrist.

Cai force. Locking the elbow.

Cai force. Locking the wrist.

Normally, after plucking or grabbing, the motion then leads either downward (as used in pick up needle from sea bottom); sideward (for example, wave hands in clouds); downward diagonally (such as diagonal flying); or upward (for instance, stand high to search out the horse). The main purpose of cai is to forcibly lead the opponent's arm in the desired direction. From this action, the opponent's balance can be destroyed, or the arm can be immobilized for further attack.

Cai applied. Downward cai used in pick up needle from the sea bottom.

Cai applied. Sideways cai used in wave hands in clouds.

Cai applied. Diagonal cai used in diagonal flying.

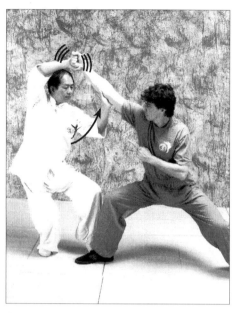

Cai applied. Upward cai used in stand high to search out the horse.

## 6. Lie (挒)

Lie force. Forward and to the side.

Lie means "to rend" or "to split." This movement has the feeling of splitting a bamboo shaft or a piece of wood into two parts. Therefore, the action is forward and to the side. Lie is the action of using the arm to split or rend so as to put your opponent into a locked position or to make him fall. Very often it is considered a sideward peng.

It can be used to lock the arm (for example, wild horses shear the mane) or to bounce the opponent off balance (as used in grasp sparrow's tail or diagonal flying).

Lie applied. Lie used in wild horses shear the mane to lock the opponent's arm.

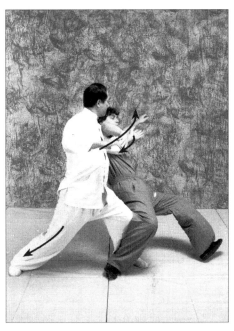

Lie applied. Lie used in grasp sparrow's tail to bounce the opponent off balance.

Lie applied. Lie used in diagonal flying to off balance the opponent.

## 7. Zhou (肘)

Zhou means "to elbow" and implies the use of the elbow to attack, or to neutralize a lock of the elbow. It includes both offensive and defensive purposes. When the elbow is used to attack through striking (*da*, 打) or pressing (ji, 擠), the chest area is the main target.

Zhou force. Striking the chest.

Zhou force. Pressing the chest.

When the elbow is used to neutralize a lock, a circular yielding motion is generally applied. From the circular yielding motion, the elbow can neutralize the attack (*hua*, 化) to wrap or coil your opponent's arm (*chan*, 纏), or to seal the opponent's arm from further attack (*feng*, 封).

Zhou force. Striking the chest.

Using the elbow to neutralize.

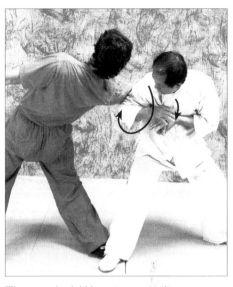

Zhou applied. Wrapping or coiling.

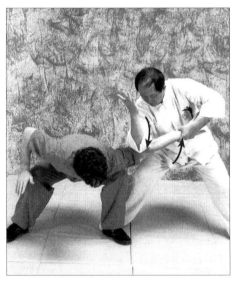

Zhou applied. Sealing the opponent's arm.

Zhou applied. Sealing the opponent's arm.

The elbow is like a steering wheel that directs its arm's movement. Therefore, it is very common that in order to immobilize your arm movement, your opponent will lock or grab your elbow, and consequently your arm will be controlled. When this happens, you must know how to circle your elbow and how to coil your forearm to reverse the situation. From this you can see that for defensive purposes, knowing how to maneuver your elbow is very important.

## 8. Kao (靠)

Kao means "to bump," and implies using part of your body, such as your shoulder (*jian kao*, 肩靠), back (*bei kao*, 背靠), hip (*tun kao*, 臀靠), thigh (*tui kao*, 腿靠), knee (*xi kao*, 膝靠), and chest (*xiong kao*, 胸靠) to bump the opponent's body.

Kao force. Using the shoulder.

Kao force. Using the back.

Kao force. Using the hip.

Kao force. Using the thigh.

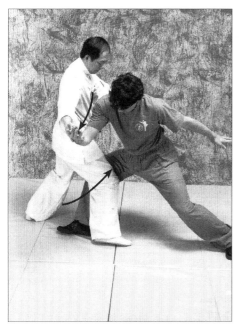

Kao force. Using the thigh.

Kao force. Using the knee.

Kao force. Using the chest.

From the direction of kao, it can be classified as forward kao (*qian kao*, 前靠), downward kao (*xia kao*, 下靠), sideways kao (*ce kao*, 側靠), and upward kao (*shang kao*, 上靠).

Kao applied. Forward.

Kao applied. Downward.

Kao applied. Sideways.

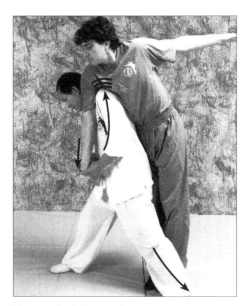

Kao applied. Upward.

Kao is especially important in very close-range situations with your opponent. If you apply kao skillfully, you can destroy your opponent's rooting and balance, and are therefore able to prevent him from further attack. Alternatively, whenever your opponent is attempting to regain his balance, you can take the opportunity to execute further action, such as kicking or striking. Naturally, you can also use kao to make your opponent fall when applied correctly. Kao is extremely powerful and destructive in some circumstances. You should be very careful in your training and should avoid using it on your opponent's vital areas, such as the solar plexus, unless you desire to cause serious injury.

## II. The Five Strategic Directional Movements

In a battle, it is very important to keep an advantageous distance between you and your opponent for your attack or defense. Because of this, all of the Chinese martial arts styles train students how to move forward, backward, and sideways for advancing, retreating, and dodging. It is the same in taijiquan. In order to apply the techniques correctly, you must know how to set up a correct distance and angle, which will allow you to have the most advantageous maneuvering. Therefore, how you step and direct your body naturally and automatically in a battle is an important factor in winning.

However, in taijiquan, due to the sticking and adhering strategy and techniques, you and your opponent are often in a stationary and urgent position. At that moment, you may not be able to step and move, since it could offer your opponent an opportunity to destroy your balance and rooting. Therefore, in taijiquan pushing hands training, stationary pushing hands has always been the first priority. In order to help you move beyond such limited training, here we will summarize the basic strategic movements in taijiquan.

### 1. Jin Bu (進步)

Step forward (jin bu, 進步) is normally used to maintain distance when your opponent is retreating. In order to stick and adhere, you must keep a good distance. Often, when your opponent realizes that your techniques are better than his, he will try to retreat and free himself from your sticking and adhering. Therefore, in order to keep him in the same awkward situation, you must know how to step forward skillfully.

Step forward is also often used to close the distance between you and your opponent from the long range into the medium or short

Jin bu (forward) stepping.

ranges, or from the medium range into the short range. For example, once you have neutralized your opponent's punch with sticking, in order to adhere to his arm, you must close from the medium range into the short range, which allows you to have better control for your taijiquan techniques. Naturally, when the opportunity allows, after you control your opponent's arms, you may step forward to gain advancing power for your striking.

Jin bu applied. First neutralize with sticking.

Then step forward to close the distance.

Jin bu applied. First control the arm.

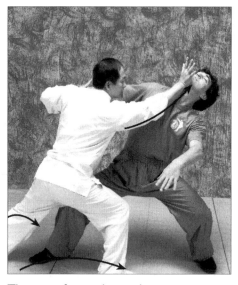

Then step forward to strike.

## 2. Tui Bu (退步)

The strategy of "step backward" is exactly opposite from that of "step forward." With stepping backward, you can retreat from an urgent situation. Often, stepping backward is used to yield to oncoming power, providing you more time to lead and neutralize an attack. For example, when your opponent is pressing your chest with his palms, you may step backward to yield and at the same time squeeze both his arms inward. From this you can see that generally speaking, "step backward" is a defensive maneuver.

Tui bu stepping.

Tui bu applied. Stepping backward for defense.

## 3. Zuo Gu (左顧)

Zuo (左) means left and gu (顧) means "see" or "look for." Therefore, zuo gu means to see or to look for the opportunity on your left. While you are in a fighting situation, you should always be looking for an opportunity to step to your sides. Stepping to the side will offer you an advantageous opportunity to enter your opponent's empty door.

Zuo gu stepping.

Often, stepping to the left is part of a technique that could put your opponent into an awkward position. For example, when you apply the large rollback (da lu, 大攦) technique, in order to make the technique effective, you must step your left leg to your left and put your opponent into a controlled position.

Zuo gu applied. Stepping to the left with the rear leg and using large rollback.

Naturally, stepping to the side is also commonly used to dodge or to avoid oncoming power. From sideways stepping, you may direct your opponent's power to the side and thereby stop him from further action. For example, in small rollback (xiao lu, 小擺), once you have neutralized your opponent's power, you may step your right leg to his right (your left) and at the same time pull him off balance.

Zou gu applied. Stepping to the left and using small rollback.

Often "zuo gu" is also translated as "beware of the left." This means to be aware of the left-side attack from your opponent. This can also be interpreted as "be aware of" an opportunity on your left.

### 4. You Pan (右盼)

This is the same strategic movement as "see the left." This time you should keep looking for an opportunity to step to your right. The purposes are the same as those of "see the left," and this technique serves for dodging and setting up advantageous angles for your attack. For example, in the large rollback (da lu, 大擺) technique, once you have performed rollback on your opponent's arm, you may step both your legs to your right; this will offer you a good angle for your pressing (ji, 擠).

You pan applied. Stepping to the right and using large rollback, and then press.

Also, in the wave hands in clouds (*yun shou*, 雲手) technique, if your opponent's left leg is forward, once you have controlled his right arm, you may step your left leg to the side of his left leg (to your right); this will offer you an advantageous angle to take him down.

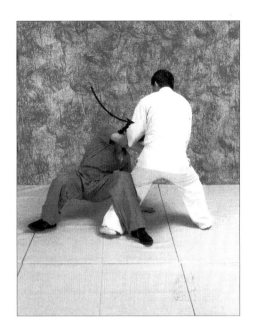

You pan applied. Stepping to the right and using wave hands in clouds.

### 5. Zhong Ding (中定)

Zhong (中) means "center" and ding (定) means "to stabilize" or "to firm." In taijiquan practice, zhong ding is probably one of the most important trainings on which a beginner should concentrate. In order to stabilize your center, you must first have a firm root. In order to have a firm root, you must first have firmed your center. In order to firm your center, you must first have good balance. In order to balance yourself, you must first know how to relax yourself and to allow the qi to move smoothly and naturally in your body. This will offer you an accurate sensation of your balance. Only if you have a firm root, then your spirit can be raised.

From this you can see that to firm the center and root is not an easy task, especially for a beginner. Generally, zhong ding is learned from standing qigong and stationary pushing hands practice. In stationary pushing hands drills, you and your partner are looking for each other's center and rooting, and trying to

Zhong ding. Firm and centered.

destroy them. Naturally, you must also learn how to protect your center and rooting from being destroyed by your partner.

## 2-4. Yi, Qi, and Action

When there is an action, we generate ideas or mind (yi, 意) first, and from this yi, the qi is led to the muscles and nerves to activate or energize the muscles for contraction and relaxation. From this you can see that the origin of any action is the yi.

Yi, or the mind, is generated within the brain. It is generally believed that we understand the functioning of only about 10 percent of the brain. From this you can see that we still cannot completely rely on modern science to explain all of the functioning or the behavior of the brain. That means our science is still in its infancy.

Except for some extraordinary people, such as Einstein or Hawking, we develop and utilize only about 33 percent of our brain. This means that about 67 percent of our brain is never even used as far as we know. Some Chinese Buddhist and Daoist qigong practices learn how to lead the qi to the brain to activate or energize the extra brain cells for functioning, and hopefully assist the practitioner to reach a stage of spiritual enlightenment.

According to the model adopted by YMAA, the qi circulating in living organisms is a form of bioelectric energy. In our analysis of this bioelectricity, it is helpful to consider that a brain cell will consume at least twelve or more times the oxygen of regular cells. Oxygen and food are the original sources of bioelectricity in the cells through biochemical reaction in the body. The twelve-fold oxygen requirements of the brain cells lead us to conclude that these cells probably consume twelve times or more electricity than ordinary cells. This means that in order to increase brain functioning to a higher level, we must learn how to charge the batteries in our body to a higher level. Only then can we hope to lead plenty of qi to the brain to activate and maintain its higher level of functioning. According to past experience with qigong practice in China, this battery is also called the *lower dan tian* (下丹田) and is located approximately at our physical center of gravity (within the large and small intestines). In order to charge the qi to a higher level in the lower dan tian, the methods of "abdominal breathing" (腹息) and "embryo breathing" (胎息) were discovered in the past. If you are interested in knowing more about these two breathing techniques, you should refer to *Tai Chi Qigong*, published by YMAA.

To lead the qi upward to the brain, concentration or meditation training is necessary. From concentration and meditation practice, the qi or bioelectricity can be led by the mind to the brain to activate more brain cells for functioning. In addition, through mind concentration, the EMF (electromotive force) generated from the brain will be stronger. Naturally, the qi or bioelectricity led or directed by the brain will be stronger.

Our physical body is like a living machine: its functioning depends on qi or bioelectricity levels. When the qi level is high, this machine can be enhanced to a higher efficiency, and when the qi level is low, the operation of the machine will be stagnant. Without special training like weightlifting or special sports, normally a person will only use less than half of his maximum physical strength for daily work. This means that unless it is necessary, most of us never demand peak functioning of our physical body.

From this you can see that in order for your body to have a higher functioning capability, you must have a concentrated, meditative mind, an abundant qi storage in the lower dan tian, and knowledge of how to lead the qi to the required body area to energize the physical body to a higher working efficiency. That is why, since AD 550, all Chinese martial styles have practiced qigong.

Some martial styles believed that since it would take a long time to develop the concentrated, meditative mind and to charge the qi in the lower dan tian to a higher level, we should first use the already available qi in our bodies to energize the physical body for fighting. It was critical that you learned techniques first for your defense in ancient times. Only after you knew how to defend yourself could you begin to cultivate your qi and train your concentrated, meditative mind. These styles are called "external styles."

However, other styles believed that since the mind and the qi are the origins of physical power, one should first learn how to cultivate the qi and train the concentrated mind. Only when the qi was strong could it be led by the concentrated mind to the physical body for techniques. In order to allow the qi to circulate smoothly in the body, the body must be soft and relaxed. This is the origin of taijiquan, known as one of the "internal styles."

From the above explanation, you can see that taijiquan emphasizes the soft and uses it against the hard. Taijiquan focuses more on internal training, such as the concentrated, meditative mind and the cultivation of qi. Finally, in order to be relaxed physically for smooth qi circulation, the movements are rounder. Not coincidentally, these same characteristics apply to qin na techniques. When you have reached the higher levels of qin na, the techniques become soft and round. The concentrated mind is the essential key to executing a technique.

## References

1. 太極拳刀、劍、桿、散手合編。陳炎林。 [Taijiquan, Saber, Sword, Staff, and Sparring] by Chen, Yan-lin, Reprinted in Taipei, Taiwan, 1943.

2. *Tai Chi Theory and Martial Power*, Dr. Yang, Jwing-Ming, YMAA, 1987.

3. 技高圈小。

# Chapter 3: Qin Na in Peng, Lu, Ji, and An

### 3-1. Introduction

As explained in the last chapter, peng, lu, ji, *an*, cai, lie, zhou, and kao are the eight fundamental methods or patterns of jing manifestation in taijiquan. From these eight patterns, hundreds of techniques can be derived and developed. Since these eight patterns are the most basic jing patterns in taijiquan, it would be wise first to understand those qin na techniques that can be applied and used against these patterns. Naturally, after you have mastered all of the qin na techniques from these eight jing patterns, you will be able to apply them into taiji pushing hands. This is because taiji pushing hands techniques are all built upon the foundation of these eight basic patterns.

In this chapter, I would like to introduce the possible qin na applications for the first four patterns: peng, lu, ji, and *an*, and in the next chapter, the remaining four patterns: cai, lie, zhou, and kao.

Again, I would like to remind you that the qin na introduced here are only some of the possible techniques with which I am familiar. Through practicing and pondering, you will soon discover there are many other techniques that can be developed according to the same theory. You should also understand that since qin na theory remains the same for any style, it is not surprising that many techniques are very similar to Shaolin Qin Na or any other style. As a matter of fact, many qin na techniques introduced in this book are adapted from Shaolin White Crane Qin Na.

### 3-2. Qin Na in Peng

Peng is expanding the chest and using the chest's arcing power to extend the arm forward, upward, or sideward. Few qin na techniques are executed using peng itself. Often it is mixed with other jing patterns such as pluck (cai, 採) or press with wrist (*an*, 按).

Normally, peng is executed with the forearm or elbow. Therefore, when you use your forearm wardoff for qin na control, you usually pay more attention to the locking of your opponent's elbow or post-arm. However, if the distance between you and your opponent is so close that you can apply peng jing to his neck, then you have the option to control his neck as well. Naturally, the same theory applies when you use qin na against peng.

## I. Qin Na for Peng

### Technique #1. Using Forearm Wardoff against the Enemy's Elbow (Bi Peng Di Zhou, 臂掤敵肘)

The *bi peng di zhou* technique is used to lock your opponent's elbow with your forearm.

Situation: Your opponent punches you with his right hand or adheres to your left arm with his right hand.

Use your left forearm to intercept or neutralize his right arm while placing your right forearm under his elbow or on the rear side of his post-arm to press his tendons.

Finally, using the leverage of your left hand and right forearm, you may lock him upward.

You may also use this leverage and jing to break his elbow. When you execute this technique, you should position yourself on your opponent's right side to avoid his left hand attack.

### Theory

Misplacing the bone (elbow) and pressing the tendon (if post-arm tendons are pressed): When you use your left forearm to neutralize the attack, you are using upward and sideways wardoff (peng) (掤) to lead and direct your opponent's oncoming force to your left. Once you have locked your opponent in the final position, you are using downward press (*an*) (按) for your left hand and upward wardoff (peng) (掤) to lock his elbow joint.

### Technique #2. Crane Spreads Its Wings or Reverse Wrist Press (Bai He Liang Chi / Fan Ya Wan, 白鶴亮翅 / 反壓腕)

The *bai he liang chi / fan ya wan* technique can be used when your opponent's right hand is either punching you or adhering to your right forearm in a pushing hands situation.

Situation: Your opponent punches you with his right fist. First, use your left forearm to cover his punching hand while at the same time clamping upward on his wrist with your right hand.

Immediately twist his wrist counterclockwise to lock it.

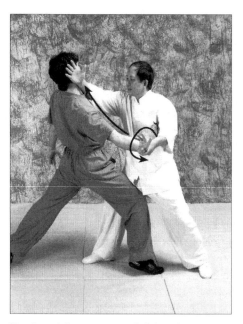

Finally, while using your left hand to continue the twisting on his right wrist, use your right forearm to push the right side of his neck.

Situation: Your opponent's right hand is adhering to your right forearm.

Use your left hand to grab his right hand.

Then twist it counterclockwise with both of your hands.

Once the position of his right arm is set, immediately use your right forearm to push the side of his neck. Using the leverage of your left hand's twisting and right forearm's pushing, you can lock him up easily.

### Theory

Misplacing the bone (elbow and shoulder) and dividing the muscle/tendon (wrist): When you grab your opponent's right wrist and twist it counterclockwise, it is a form of pluck (cai, 採). When you use your right forearm to push his neck, it is a sideways peng. In this technique, you should pay attention to the angle at which you lock his right arm. If his arm is either too straight or too bent, the technique will not be effective. Naturally, your right arm's wardoff also plays a main role in the locking. With an accurate wardoff angle of your right arm, you may generate effective leverage for your locking.

## Technique #3. Upward Elbow Wrap (Shang Chan Zhou, 上纏肘)

Although the *shang chan zhou* technique is very similar to the bai he liang chi / fan ya wan technique, the means of approaching and locking are somewhat different.

Situation: Your opponent's right hand is adhering to your right wrist.

After you have neutralized his power to your right, use your left hand to grab his right hand.

Twist his hand counterclockwise with both of your hands.

Next, reposition yourself to his right side, continue twisting his right wrist with your left hand while coiling your right hand around his right arm, and reach to his elbow and lift it upward. In this case, you have used the leverage of your left and right hands to lock his right arm.

In order to control him more effectively, you may lock his right arm with your right hand and right abdominal area while using your left forearm to push his neck or head sideways or forward.

## Theory

Misplacing the bone (elbow and shoulder): Again, the left hand's grabbing is a form of pluck (cai, 採). Your right hand's coiling and reaching to his elbow is a jing of coiling (chan, 纏), and in the final position of locking, your left forearm's pushing and expanding is a form of sideways wardoff or forward wardoff (peng, 掤). To make this technique effective, you should raise his right elbow high with your right hand while pushing away his neck or head with your left forearm. Remember when you apply your qin na technique to be soft, easy, and circular. This will prevent your opponent from feeling your intention before you lock him.

## Technique #4. Prop Up Elbow (Shang Jia Zhou, 上架肘)

The *shang jia zhou* technique is for when your opponent's right hand is adhering to your right wrist.

Situation: Your opponent's right hand is adhering to your right wrist.

Reposition yourself to his right side, coil your right hand counterclockwise around his forearm, and then either press it down or grab his wrist while placing your left hand on his elbow to stop him from elbowing you.

Next, place your left elbow under his right elbow and use the leverage of your right hand and left elbow to straighten his right arm and lift him upward. The internal side of his arm should face upward.

Finally, use the right hand's pressing and the left post-arm's upward wardoff power to generate leverage and lock him upward.

**Theory**

Misplacing the bone (elbow): When you circle your right hand around his forearm and finally reach his wrist, it is a form of coiling (chan, 纏). In the final locking, if you use your right hand to press his wrist down, it is a downward press (*an*), and if your right hand is used to lock or grab his wrist, then it is a pluck (cai, 採). Naturally, your left post-arm's upward lifting and expanding is an upward wardoff (peng, 掤) generated from your left post-arm. In this technique, you may also use your post-arm to press the rear tendons of his post-arm upward. If you do so, then it is a mixture of the body misplacing the bone (elbow) and pressing the tendon (post-arm) techniques.

### Technique #5. Crane Spreads Its Wings (Bai He Liang Chi, 白鶴亮翅)

Use bai he liang chi when your opponent's left hand is adhering to your right wrist or forearm.

Situation: Your opponent's left hand is adhering to your right wrist or forearm.

First, raise your right arm and use your left hand to grab his left hand.

Next, twist his left wrist with both of your hands, circling his arm downward clockwise.

Finally, step both of your legs forward to shorten the distance between you and your opponent while locking his left arm by your stomach and using your right forearm to push his chin upward and forward.

## Theory

Misplacing the bone (elbow and shoulder) and dividing the muscle/tendon (wrist): This is again an application of the taijiquan posture the crane spreads its wings. Your left hand's grabbing is a form of pluck (cai) and your right forearm's pushing and expanding is a form of sideways wardoff (peng, 掤). The leverage generated from your left hand's twisting and your right forearm's expanding wardoff jing is the key to the locking.

### Technique #6. Using Arm Wardoff against the Enemy's Leg (Bi Peng Di Tui, 臂掤敵腿)

Use *bi peng di tui* when both of your arms are wide open.

Situation: During pushing hands, when both of your arms are wide open, it is possible for your opponent to kick you.

If your opponent kicks your middle body with his right leg, immediately use your left forearm to scoop his right leg upward.

Finally, use your right hand to press his toes downward while lifting your left forearm onto the tendons of his calf.

## Theory

Pressing the tendon (calf): This is an example of upward wardoff (peng, 掤) against a kick. After you have scooped his leg and trapped it, the upward wardoff jing must be strong, simply because his leg is also strong. If your left arm is right on his calf tendons, with the leverage generated from your left forearm and right hand's downward pressing (an, 按), you can create great pain in his calf. You should keep his leg as straight as possible. That means you may have to raise his leg higher.

## II. Qin Na against Peng

### Technique #1. Small Elbow Wrap (Xiao Chan Zhou, 小纏肘)

Use the *xiao chan zhou* technique when your opponent is using his forearm to perform upward or forward wardoff against your chest.

Situation: Your opponent is using his forearm to perform upward or forward wardoff against your chest.

First, use your right forearm to raise his right forearm while placing your left hand on his elbow.

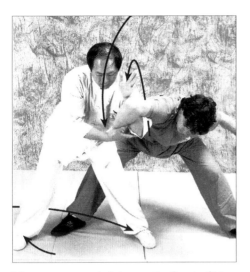

Next, step your left leg to the front of his right leg, grab his right wrist with your right hand, and use the leverage of your left forearm and right hand to rotate his right arm.

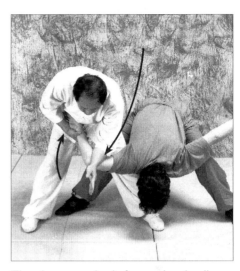

Then bow your body forward and pull his body toward your front to destroy his balance.

Finally, sweep your left leg backward to take him down.

If you like, you may use both of your legs to lock his arm behind him while using your hands to grab his hair to control him completely.

## Theory

Misplacing the bone (shoulder): The first movement in which you use your right forearm to lead his arm upward is an upward wardoff (peng, 掤). When you circle his arm downward, it is a downward rollback (lu, 攦). Naturally, your right hand's grabbing is a pluck (cai, 採). The trick to making this technique successful is to lead your opponent to your front; this will destroy his balance for your sweeping.

## Technique #2. Old Man Carries the Fish on His Back (Lao Han Bei Yu, 老漢背魚)

You can use the *lao han bei yu* technique if your opponent is using his right forearm to perform wardoff against your chest, either forward or upward.

Situation: Your opponent is using his right forearm to perform wardoff against your chest, either forward or upward.

Immediately use your left forearm to push his elbow downward while using your right hand to raise his forearm to bend his arm.

Finally, step your left leg behind him, turn your body to your right, and then bow forward to lock his right arm behind your back.

### Theory

Misplacing the bone (shoulder and elbow): When you use both of your arms to bend his elbow, it is an action of squeezing (ji, 擠) like the posture of play the guitar in taijiquan. In the final position of locking, it is using the back upward pressing (kao, 靠) to set up a locking angle. To make this technique effective, your opponent's arm should not be too bent or too straight.

**Technique #3. Upward Wrist Press (Shang Ya Wan, 上壓腕)**

Use *shang ya wan* if your opponent uses his right arm to perform wardoff against your chest, either forward or upward.

Situation: Your opponent uses his right arm to perform wardoff against your chest, either forward or upward.

Immediately use your right hand to grab his right wrist while placing your left hand on his elbow and pushing it upward.

Finally, move your left leg closer to your right leg, pressing your right hand upward to generate strain on his wrist while pressing your left hand downward on his elbow. This will generate leverage for the locking. You should increase your squeezing pressure until his heels are off the ground.

**Theory**

Dividing the muscle/tendon (wrist): Again, when using both of your hands to control his wrist and elbow, it is an action of squeeze (ji, 擠). This kind of squeezing motion is also called close (*he*, 合) in taijiquan. Naturally, the right hand's grabbing is an action of pluck (cai, 採). Once you have locked his arm upward, the final lock is generated from the squeeze (ji, 擠) of both hands.

### Technique #4. Press Shoulder with Single Finger / Extending the Neck for Water (Yi Zhi Ding Jian / Yin Jing Qiu Shui, 一指頂肩 / 引頸求水

Use *yi zhi ding jian / yin jing qiu shui* when your opponent uses his forearm to perform wardoff against your chest.

Situation: Your opponent uses his forearm to perform wardoff against your chest.

First, use your right hand to grab his wrist while using your left forearm to press his elbow upward.

Next, step your left leg behind his right leg, coil your left hand around his right arm until your left hand reaches his post-arm near the elbow, and lift your left elbow to lock his arm behind him.

Jianneiling
(M-UE-48)

In this case, the shoulder area ligaments will be very tensed. If you use your index or middle finger to press his *jianneiling* (M-UE-48, 肩內陵) cavity upward, you will be able to generate great pain in his shoulder.

Alternatively, you may use your hand to press his chin upward to generate leverage for locking.

## Theory

Misplacing the bone (shoulder) and cavity press (jianneiling cavity, 肩內陵): Again, your right hand's grabbing is a pluck (cai, 採), and both hands' closing and rotating movements are actions of squeeze (ji, 擠) or close (he, 合). Circling your left hand around his right arm until the post-arm near the elbow is an action of coil (chan, 纏), and when you lift up your elbow while pressing your left hand on his post-arm, it is a downward press (an, 按). Naturally, in the final locking, your right hand's lifting is a raise or lift (ti, 提), and when you use your finger to press his jianneiling cavity (M-UE-48, 肩內陵), it is a point or press (dian, 點).

**Technique #5. Reverse Elbow Wrap (Fan Chan Zhou, 反纏肘)**

Strictly speaking, the *fan chan zhou* technique is an option of the previous yi zhi ding jian / yin jing qiu shui technique.

Situation: Your opponent uses his right forearm to perform wardoff against your chest.

First, step your left leg behind his right leg, grabbing his right wrist with your right hand while coiling your left hand around his arm until it reaches his post-arm near the elbow.

Next, lift his forearm upward with your left elbow while stepping your right leg backward.

Finally, circle him down to the ground.

**Theory**

Misplacing the bone (shoulder): Again, your right hand's grabbing is a pluck (cai, 採) and your left hand's circling around his right arm until the post-arm is near the elbow is an action of coil (chan, 纏). When you lift up your elbow while pressing your left hand on his post-arm to generate strain on his shoulder, it is a downward press (*an*, 按). Finally, the action of leading him to the ground is a movement of rollback (lu, 攌).

## Technique #6. Upward Elbow Wrap (Shang Chan Zhou, 上纏肘)

Use shang chan zhou when your opponent uses his right forearm to perform wardoff against your chest.

Situation: Your opponent uses his right forearm to perform wardoff against your chest.

Use your left forearm to press his elbow down while using your right forearm to raise his right forearm.

Next, circle his arm counterclockwise while grabbing his wrist with your left hand.

Continue the circular motion of both of your hands, and then twist his wrist with your left hand while pressing his elbow upward with your right hand.

To make the lock more effective, you should squeeze both of your hands toward each other. Alternatively, you may lock his right arm with your right hand and abdominal area while using your left hand to push his head either sideward or forward.

**Theory**

Misplacing the bone (shoulder and elbow): Your left hand's grabbing on his wrist is a pluck (cai, 採), and the circling of your right hand around his arm until his elbow is a coil (chan, 纏). When you squeeze both hands toward each other, it is a squeeze (ji, 擠), and your left forearm's pushing against his neck or head is a wardoff (peng, 掤). Remember that the circular motions in taijiquan are very important. It is the same in taiji qin na. When you use circular motions, you are able to set up a qin na lock before your opponent feels it. A good qin na technique is soft, smooth, and round. The action should be natural, easy, and straightforward.

## 3-3. Qin Na in Lu

As explained in chapter 2, lu means to yield, lead, and then neutralize to the side and backward; it is commonly translated as "rollback." Lu is generally used for defensive purposes. However, when the situation is right, lu can be used to attack. In this section, we will introduce the offensive lu, which can be used for qin na. Then we will review some of the qin na that can be used against lu.

### I. Qin Na for Lu

When you use lu to yield, lead, control, or neutralize the opponent's arm, normally you use one hand to grab or pluck your opponent's wrist while using the other hand to control his elbow or post-arm. Lu can be distinguished as "small rollback" and "large rollback."

### Technique #1. Large Rollback (Da Lu, 大攦)

Use da lu when your opponent's hands are on your right forearm, either pushing it or pressing it downward.

Situation. Your opponent's hands are on your right forearm, either pushing it or pressing it downward.

First, step your right leg backward to yield and lead, neutralizing his power backward by grabbing his right wrist with your right hand and placing your left forearm on his post-arm or elbow.

Finally, step your right leg back and use the leverage generated from both of your hands to lock his arm and lead him down to the ground.

**Theory**

Misplacing the bone (elbow) or press the tendon (post-arm): Your right hand's grabbing is a pluck (cai, 採). In fact, the entire motion is a large rollback (da lu, 大擺). If you use your left forearm to press the tendons in his post-arm, the location of pressing is important. The place to press is about three inches above the elbow.

**Technique #2. Lead the Snake to Enter the Cave (Yin She Ru Dong, 引蛇入洞)**

Use *yin she ru dong* when both of your opponent's hands are on your right forearm.

Situation: Both of your opponent's hands are on your right forearm.

First, apply wardoff against his power while using your left hand to grab his left wrist.

Next, coil your right hand around his left arm until you reach his elbow, and lock his arm straight.

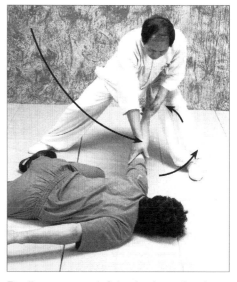

Finally, step your left leg backward and use the leverage of both of your hands to lead him down to the ground.

## Theory

Misplacing the bone (elbow): The entire action is the technique of small rollback (xiao lu, 小擺). When you raise your right arm upward, it is an upward wardoff (peng, 掤); when you circle your right hand around his left arm until you reach his elbow, it is a coil (chan, 纏). The left hand's wrist grabbing is a pluck (cai, 採), and naturally, when you lead his power to the ground, it is rollback (lu, 擺).

### Technique #3. Hands Hold a Panda (Shou Bao Wan Xiong, 手抱浣熊)

Use *shou bao wan xiong* when both of your opponent's hands are on your right forearm. First, use upward wardoff against the oncoming power.

Situation: Your opponent's hands are on your right forearm. First, use wardoff upward against the oncoming power.

Next, coil your right hand around his right arm until it reaches the internal side of his elbow while also using your left hand to grab his right wrist and circle his arm downward.

Then step your right leg behind his right leg while pulling his right elbow in with your right hand. And using your left hand, push his right wrist to his back.

Finally, use your right hand and your chest to lock his arm behind him and use your left hand to push his chin away.

## Theory

Dividing the muscle/tendon (wrist): When you raise your right arm upward, it is an upward wardoff (peng, 掤). When you circle your right hand around his right arm, it is a coil (chan, 纏). The left hand's grabbing is a pluck (cai), and when you lead his power to your left and backward, it is a small rollback (xiao lu, 小攦). Finally, when you lock his right arm between your right hand and chest, it is a squeeze (ji, 擠).

### Technique #4. Small Elbow Wrap (Xiao Chan Zhou, 小纏肘)

Use xiao chan zhou when your opponent's hands are on your right forearm and are pressing.

Situation: Your opponent's hands are pressing on your right forearm.

First, raise your right arm in an upward wardoff against his power and grab his right wrist while also placing your left forearm on his right elbow and circling his arm downward. Right after you neutralize his power, you should immediately step your left leg to the front of his right leg.

Finally, lead his arm and body to the front of your body while sweeping your left leg backward to make him fall.

## Theory

Misplacing the bone (shoulder and elbow): Your right arm's raising is an upward wardoff (peng, 掤) and its grabbing is a pluck (cai, 採). When you lead his body to your front and make him fall, it is a rollback (lu, 攦).

## Technique #5. Reverse Elbow Wrap (Fan Chan Zhou, 反纏肘)

Use fan chan zhou when both of your opponent's hands are on your right forearm and ready to press down.

Situation: Your opponent's hands are on your right forearm and ready to press down.

Immediately step your left leg behind his right leg and raise your right arm to an upward wardoff against the power. Next, grab his wrist while coiling your left hand around his right arm until it reaches his post-arm near the elbow. Then lock his arm behind his back.

Finally, step your right leg backward while leading him down to the ground.

The locking leverage is generated from your left elbow and hand.

## Theory

Misplacing the bone (shoulder and elbow): When you raise your right arm to neutralize his pressing, it is an upward wardoff (peng, 掤), and then its grabbing on his right wrist is a pluck (cai, 採). When you circle your left hand around his right arm, it is a coil (chan, 纏), and finally when you lead him down to the ground, it is a rollback (lu, 攦).

### Technique #6. Push the Boat to Follow the Stream (Shun Shui Tui Zhou, 順水推舟)

Use *shun shui tui zhou* when your opponent's left hand is on your right wrist.

Situation: Your opponent's left hand is on your right wrist.

Immediately turn your right hand upward and circle around his wrist while using your left hand to grab his left wrist.

Next, step your left leg backward and twist his wrist with your left hand while using your right hand, which is on his wrist, to control his left arm.

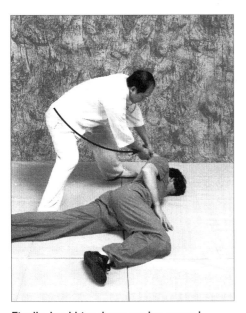

Finally, lead him down to the ground.

The control is generated from twisting the wrist of his left hand.

## Theory

Dividing the muscle/tendon (wrist): Your right hand's circling around his left wrist is a coil (chan, 纏) and your left hand's grabbing is a pluck (cai, 採). When you lead his body down to the ground, it is a rollback (lu, 攦). The key control of this technique is on the twisting of his wrist with your left hand. Your right hand is only to help you control his arm.

### Technique #7. Wild Chicken Breaks Its Wings (Ye Ji Yao Chi, 野雞拗翅)

Use *ye ji yao chi* when your opponent's right hand is pressing or pushing your chest.

 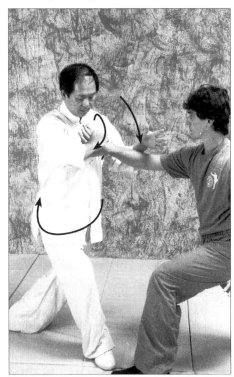

Situation: Your opponent's right hand is pressing or pushing your chest.

Immediately turn your body to your right. Use your right hand to grab his right wrist and turn it clockwise ninety degrees while placing your left hand on his elbow.

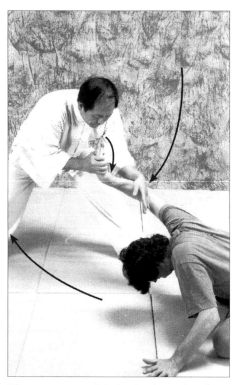

Then step your right leg backward and at the same time use the leverage generated from both of your hands to press him downward.

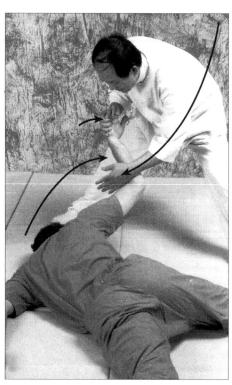

You may continue your locking pressure and lead him until his entire body is on the ground.

## Theory

Dividing the muscle/tendon (wrist): When you use your right hand to grab his right wrist, it is a pluck (cai, 採), and when you lead him down to the ground, it is a rollback (lu, 挒). In this technique, when you control your opponent, his elbow should be lower than his wrist. The entire control is on the twisting and bending of his wrist by your right hand. Your left hand only serves to keep his elbow down.

**Technique #8. Arm Rolls Back the Enemy's Elbow (Bi Lu Di Zhou, 臂攄敵肘)**

Use *bi lu di zhou* to control your opponent's right hand when he places it on your left shoulder.

Situation: Your opponent's right hand is on your left shoulder. To control it, immediately turn your body to your right to yield.

Next, use your right hand to grab his right wrist while placing your left forearm on his right elbow.

Finally, step your right leg backward, bow toward him, and use the leverage of both of your hands to lead him down.

You may continue to step your right leg backward to lead him down to the ground.

### Theory

Dividing the muscle/tendon (wrist): When you use your right hand to grab his right wrist, it is a pluck (cai, 採), and when you lead him down to the ground, it is a rollback (lu, 攦). In this technique, when you control your opponent, his elbow should be lower than his wrist. The entire control is on his wrist's twisting and bending by your right hand. Your left forearm only serves to keep his elbow down.

## II. Qin Na against Lu

When your opponent uses "small rollback" against you, one of his hands will be grabbing your wrist while the other leads and controls your elbow joint to rollback. When your opponent uses the "large rollback" while one of his hands is grabbing you, the forearm of the other arm will be on your elbow or post-arm area.

It is not easy to grab your opponent's forearm that is on your elbow or post-arm. Therefore, there are not many qin na you can use against his forearm's rollback. However, in order to make the rollback technique effective, your opponent must use the other hand to pluck your wrist. This will offer you many options for qin na techniques to use against his pluck (cai, 採). We will examine the qin na against pluck in the next chapter. In this section, we will introduce some of the possible qin na techniques that can be used against lu.

### Technique #1. Send the Devil to Heaven (Song Mo Shang Tian, 送魔上天)

Use *song mo shang tian* when your opponent uses the small rollback technique to control your right arm and intends to lead it to his side.

Situation: Your opponent uses the small rollback technique to control your right arm and intends to lead it to his side. Immediately use your left hand to grab his right hand.

Next, step your left leg behind your right leg while twisting his right wrist with your left hand, and free your right arm through the gap of his thumb and index finger.

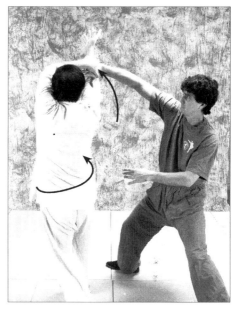

Then turn your body counterclockwise while lifting his right arm.

Continue to turn your body and twist his wrist with both hands.

Finally, lock his arm upward until his heels are off the ground.

## Theory

Dividing the muscle/tendon (wrist): Your left hand grabbing is a pluck (cai, 採), and the final twisting on his wrist is a turning (*zhuan*, 轉). To make this technique most effective, you should use your left hand to twist his wrist while using your right hand to grab his fingers and bend them downward.

### Technique #2. Forward Upward Turning (Qian Shang Fan, 前上翻)

Use *qian shang fan* when your opponent is leading your right arm to your right with a small rollback.

Situation: Your opponent is leading your right arm to your right with a small rollback.

Immediately use your left hand to grab his right wrist and circle it up while stepping your left leg behind him.

When you do this, you should use your left elbow to push his elbow to keep his arm bent. Next, reposition yourself and use both hands to bend his right arm backward.

Finally, let your right hand take over the control and use your left hand to push the upper back of his head to lock him in place.

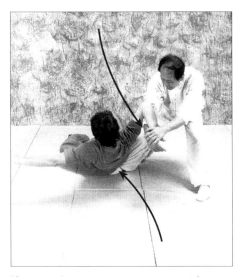

If you wish, you may sweep your right leg backward while pulling his right arm backward to take him down.

## Theory

Misplacing the bone (shoulder and elbow): At the beginning, your left hand grabbing is a pluck (cai, 採). When you step your left leg behind him and use your elbow to push his elbow to keep it bent, it is an elbow leaning against push (kao, 靠). When you push both of your hands down against his forearm to keep it bent, it is a press down (an, 按), and the final position of control is a rend (lie, 挒). You should remember that the stepping of your legs is coordinated with the technique, instead of the technique coordinating with the steppings. Therefore, you should always look for better stepping that offers you a better position for controlling.

### Technique #3. Old Man Carries the Fish on His Back (Lao Han Bei Yu, 老漢背魚)

The lao han bei yu technique is also used against a small rollback. Though it is similar, the theory of locking is different.

Situation: Your opponent is leading your right arm to his left with both hands.

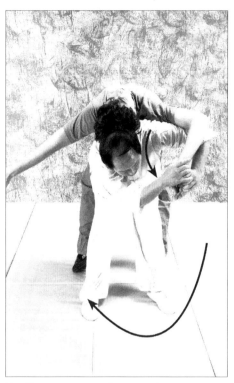

Step your left leg behind his right leg, use your left hand to grab his right wrist, and use your left elbow to push against his elbow to keep it bent.

Finally, step your right leg and pull his arm backward while bowing forward and using your upper back to push against his upper back.

## Theory

Misplacing the bone (shoulder and elbow): At the beginning, your left hand grabbing is a pluck (cai, 採). When you step your left leg behind him and use your elbow to push his elbow to keep it bent, it is an elbow leaning against push (kao, 靠). Finally, when using your upper back to push his upper back, it is a lean against (kao, 靠). When you control your opponent in the final position, his arm should not be too bent or too straight. A ninety-degree angle in the elbow is the most effective setup.

## Technique #4. Feudal Lord Lifts the Tripod (Ba Wang Tai Ding, 霸王抬鼎)

*Ba wang tai ding* is a technique against a small rollback in which your opponent is trying to lock your elbow.

Situation: Your opponent tries to lock your left arm with both of his hands.

Immediately scoop up your left elbow to prevent him from locking you, and use your right hand to grab his right wrist.

Next, reposition yourself, free your left hand, and then push his elbow to your right while twisting his right wrist to keep his arm bent.

Finally, continue your right hand twisting on his wrist while lifting and squeezing his elbow toward your right hand with your left hand to lock him in position.

### Theory

Dividing the muscle/tendon (wrist) and misplacing the bone (elbow): Your right hand's grabbing is a pluck (cai, 採), and when you raise your left arm up to neutralize his grabbing, it is a wardoff (peng, 掤). In the final lock, it is a squeeze (ji, 擠). Remember, where you stand is very important. Your final position should be far beyond his left hand's reach.

### Technique #5. Crane Spreads Its Wings and Arm Wraps Around the Dragon's Neck (Bai He Liang Chi / Bi Chan Long Jing, 白鶴亮翅 / 臂纏龍頸)

*Bai he liang chi / bi chan long jing* is again used against small rollback on your arm.

Situation: Your opponent's two hands are leading your left arm to his left.

Scoop your left arm upward to prevent your opponent from locking you, and use your right hand to grab his right wrist.

Next, reposition yourself, twist his left wrist with your right hand, and lock his arm on your stomach while placing your left elbow on his throat.

Finally, increase your right hand's twisting and pulling backward to generate pain in his left arm while expanding your left arm against his throat to lock him.

Alternatively, you may continue extending your left arm around his neck and lock his neck in place.

### Theory

Dividing the muscle/tendon (wrist), misplacing the bone (elbow), and sealing the breath (neck in alternative technique): Your left arm's upward scooping is an upward wardoff (peng, 掤), and your right hand's grabbing is a pluck (cai, 採). When you expand your left arm to lock his neck, it is also a wardoff (peng, 掤), while your locking of his arm with your stomach is a lean against (kao, 靠) with the stomach area. When you circle your left arm around his neck, it is a coil (chan, 纏).

### Technique #6. White Crane Twists Its Neck (Bai He Niu Jing, 白鶴扭頸)

The *bai he niu jing* technique is used against a large rollback.

Situation: Your opponent's right hand is grabbing your right wrist while his left forearm is on your right post-arm, getting ready to lead you down.

Immediately use your left hand to grab his left fingers.

Next, twist his fingers toward him to generate pain in the base of his pinkie tendons.

Finally, free your right hand and press his elbow downward while continuing the twisting of his fingers to lock his left arm. You should lead him down to the ground.

## Theory

Dividing the muscle/tendon (base of pinkie): Your left hand grabbing is a pluck (cai, 採), and the final twisting of his fingers is a turning (zhuan, 轉). The force of squeezing from both hands is a squeeze (ji, 擠). To make this technique most effective, you should place your mind and attention on the base of his pinkie. When your mind is there, you will be able to feel the locking easily.

## Technique #7. Play the Guitar (Shou Hui Pi Po, 手揮琵琶)

The *shou hui pi po* technique is used against the large rollback.

Situation: Your opponent's right hand is grabbing your right wrist while his left forearm is on your post-arm.

Use your left hand to grab his left fingers.

Next, twist his fingers toward him and then circle downward while using your right hand to push his elbow upward.

Finally, raise both of your hands and use the leverage of both hands to lock him in place.

It is very important that you twist his fingers in the correct angle, one that allows you to lock his pinkie's tendon on the base of the finger.

## Theory

Dividing the muscle/tendon (base of pinkie): Your left hand grabbing is a pluck (cai, 採), the final twisting on his fingers is a turning (zhuan, 轉), and the force of squeezing from both hands is a squeeze (ji, 擠). To make this technique most effective, you should place your mind and attention on the base of his pinkie. When your mind is there, you will be able to feel the locking easily.

### Technique #8. White Crane Bores the Bush (Bai He Chuan Cong, 白鶴穿叢)

The *bai he chuan cong* technique can be considered as an option to the shou hui pi pa technique. However, the locking theory is different.

Situation: Your opponent uses his right hand to grab your right wrist while using his left forearm to press your post-arm. Use your left hand to grab his left fingers.

Immediately twist his fingers to lock the tendons on the base of his pinkie while freeing your right hand, and push his left elbow upward.

Finally, circle his arm to his back and sandwich his arm between your left hand and chest while using your right hand to pull his hair backward.

## Theory

Dividing the muscle/tendon (base of pinkie): Your left hand grabbing is a pluck (cai, 採), and the final locking of his arm with your left hand and chest is a squeeze (ji, 擠). To make this technique most effective, after you have locked his hand behind him, you should put more pressure toward his pinkie to generate pain in the pinkie's tendons. To prevent him from struggling, your right hand pulling of his hair is important. This action can destroy his balance and stability, which is necessary to prevent strong struggling.

## Technique #9. Left Right Cross Elbow (Zuo You Jiao Zhou, 左右交肘)

Use *zuo you jiao zhou* when your opponent's right hand is grabbing your right wrist while his left forearm is on your post-arm.

Situation: Your opponent's right hand is grabbing your right wrist while his left forearm is on your post-arm. First, use your left hand to grab his left wrist.

Next, bend your right elbow and grab his right wrist with your right hand while pulling his left hand toward his right.

Finally, twist both of his arms and lock them in place. His left arm should be straight.

**Theory**

Misplacing the bone (elbow): Your left hand grabbing is a pluck (cai, 採), and the final twisting of his arms is a turning (zhuan, 轉). To make this technique most effective, you should use his right arm to push against his left elbow and keep it straight.

## 3-4. Qin Na in Ji

As mentioned in chapter 2, ji means to squeeze or to press, which can be done by two hands or the arms squeezing against each other. It can also be executed by pressing forward with two hands, one hand and one forearm, or even two forearms.

### I. Qin Na for Ji

Ji is normally used for offense. However, it can be used for defense when the situation is right. For example, when your opponent uses his two hands to "stamp" or "press" (an, 按) your chest, you may use both of your hands to squeeze his elbows to the center and downward to neutralize his an. Honestly speaking, there are not too many qin na techniques that use forward ji. However, there are many techniques where the ji is done by pressing both hands against each other. In this section, we will introduce some of the possible ji qin na in taijiquan.

Situation: Your opponent uses *an* to stamp or press your chest.

Neutralizing *an* with ji.

**Technique #1. Two Hands Squeeze the Wrist (Shuang Shou Ji Wan, 雙手擠腕)**

Use *shuang shou ji wan* when both of your hands are on your opponent's wrist and elbow joints.

Situation: Your hands are on your opponent's wrist and elbow joints.

Immediately use your right hand to grab his right wrist and bend it downward while using your left hand to grab his right arm and squeeze it inward to generate proper leverage for your right hand's wrist locking.

You should position yourself on his right side to avoid his left hand attack.

**Theory**

Dividing the muscle/tendon (wrist): Your right hand grabbing is a pluck (cai, 採), and the final squeezing action is a squeeze (ji, 擠). Occasionally, you will encounter an opponent who is extremely flexible. In this case, this technique will not be effective. If you realize this, immediately use your right leg or knee to strike his groin.

**Technique #2. Upward, Horizontal, and Downward Wrist Press (Shang, Zhong, Xia Ya Wan, 上，中，下壓腕)**

Use *shang, zhong, xia ya wan* when both of your hands are on your opponent's wrist and elbow joints.

Situation: Your hands are on your opponent's wrist and elbow joints.

Immediately bend his wrist inward and then upward while using your left hand to squeeze his elbow downward to generate proper leverage for your right hand's wrist locking.

Alternatively, you may lock his arm in front of your chest.

Or even squeeze his arm in front of your abdominal area.

## Theory

Dividing the muscle/tendon (wrist): Your right hand grabbing is a pluck (cai, 採), and the final squeezing action is a squeeze (ji, 擠). Occasionally, you will encounter an opponent who is extremely flexible. In this case, this technique will not be effective. If you realize this, immediately use your right leg or knee to strike his groin.

**Technique #3. Both Hands Seize the Murderer (Shuang Shou Qin Xiong, 雙手擒凶)**

Use *shuang shou qin xiong* when both of your opponent's hands are on your right forearm.

Situation: Both of your opponent's hands are on your right forearm. First, turn to your right to neutralize his pressing or pushing.

Next, immediately reposition yourself and use your right hand to grab his right wrist while coiling your left hand around his right arm until it reaches his post-arm near the elbow, and lock his arm behind him.

Finally, use your right hand to push his shoulder upward while squeezing your left hand downward and lifting your left elbow upward to lock him.

## Theory

Misplacing the bone (shoulder): Your right hand's grabbing is a pluck (cai, 採), your left hand's circling around his right arm up to his post-arm is a coil (chan, 纏), and both hands' squeezing is a squeeze (ji, 擠). In this technique, to prevent his right arm from straightening out, you must use your left elbow to lock his right forearm. In order to make the pain significant, you must raise his right arm up with your left arm.

### Technique #4. Squeeze to Seal the Breath (Ji Xiong Bi Qi, 擠胸閉氣)

Use *ji xiong bi qi* when both of your opponent's hands are on your right forearm.

Situation: Both of your opponent's hands are on your right forearm.

Step your right leg back and your left leg behind him to neutralize his pressing or pushing while covering with your left forearm on his elbow.

Next, continue to coil your left hand around his right arm. Finally, reach the back of his upper chest to squeeze forward, and at the same time squeeze your right hand toward his solar plexus to seal his breath.

## Theory

Sealing the breath (solar plexus): Your left hand's circling around your opponent's right arm is a coil (chan, 纏), and the final pressing action of both hands is a squeeze (ji, 擠).

## Technique #5. Upward Elbow Wrap (Shang Chan Zhou, 上纏肘)

Use shang chan zhou when both of your opponent's hands are on your right forearm.

Situation: Both of your opponent's hands are on your right forearm.

Immediately reposition yourself behind his right leg while using your left hand to grab his right wrist.

Next, coil your right hand around his right arm until it reaches his elbow. Finally, use the leverage generated from both hands to lock him upward.

In order to make this technique effective, you should strongly twist his right wrist with your left hand while squeezing his post-arm toward you to generate the correct leverage for locking.

### Theory

Dividing the muscle/tendon (wrist): Your left hand's grabbing is a pluck (cai, 採), the final twisting of his wrist is a turning (zhuan, 轉), and the locking generated from both hands' pressing is a squeeze (ji, 擠). To make this technique most effective, you should use your left hand to twist his wrist strongly while squeezing your right hand inward to generate good leverage.

### II. Qin Na against Ji

Other than qin na, in actual taijiquan applications, there are not too many occasions in which ji is executed by squeezing both hands against each other. Ji is done more often by pressing forward. In this section, we will focus on qin na that can be applied to this forward pressing.

As mentioned earlier, when ji is executed by pressing forward, normally your opponent uses both of his hands, one hand and one forearm, or both forearms to press forward. Generally speaking, the best option against these kinds of ji is to lock his elbow or shoulder.

### Technique #1. Old Man Carries the Fish on His Back (Lao Han Bei Yu, 老漢背魚)

Use lao han bei yu when your opponent uses both of his hands to press your chest.

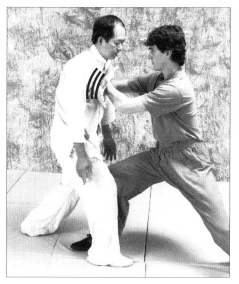

Situation: Your opponent uses both of his hands to press your chest.

Immediately use your right hand to raise his right forearm while using your left forearm to press his right elbow downward.

Next, use both of your hands to lock his right forearm while stepping your left leg behind his right leg.

Finally, bow forward and pull his arm down to lock him behind your back.

## Theory

Misplacing the bone (shoulder and elbow): Your both forearms' intercepting his right arm is an action of squeeze (ji, 擠), and in the final position of locking, it is the back lean against (kao, 靠). In order to make this technique effective, you must keep his arm bent. The best locking angle for his forearm and post-arm is at ninety degrees.

### Technique #2. Press Shoulder with Single Finger / Extending the Neck for Water (Yi Zhi Ding Jian / Yin Jing Qiu Shui, 一指頂肩 / 引頸求水)

Use yi zhi ding jian / yin jing qiu shui when your opponent presses your chest with both of his hands.

Situation: Your opponent presses your chest with both of his hands.

Immediately use your right hand to grab his right wrist while pushing his right elbow upward with your left hand.

Next, reposition yourself while coiling your left hand around his right arm until it reaches his post-arm near the elbow to lock his arm behind him. Under these conditions, the tendon in his shoulder should be very tensed.

If you press your index or middle finger upward into his jianneiling cavity (M-UE-48), significant pain can be generated.

Alternatively, you may use your right hand to raise his chin to generate more leverage.

## Theory

Misplacing the bone (shoulder) and cavity press (jianneiling cavity, 肩內陵): At the beginning, your right hand's grabbing is a pluck (cai, 採), your left hand's circling around his arm is a coil (chan, 纏), and the final cavity press is a point (dian, 點). His arm locked behind him should be kept bent. The trick of doing this is to use your left elbow to prevent him from straightening his arm.

### Technique #3. Large Wrap Hand (Do Chan Shou, 大纏手)

Use *do chan shou* when your opponent presses your chest with both of his hands.

Situation: Your opponent presses your chest with both of his hands.

Immediately scoop your right arm upward to neutralize his pressing while grabbing his right wrist with your left hand.

Next, reposition yourself, coil your right hand around his right arm until it reaches his post-arm near the elbow, and use the leverage generated from both hands to press him downward.

You may circle to your right to force him to the ground.

## Theory

Misplacing the bone (shoulder and elbow): Your right forearm's upward scooping is a wardoff (peng) (掤). Your left hand's grabbing is a pluck (cai, 採), your right hand's coiling is a coil (chan, 纏), and your right hand's downward pressing is a press (an, 按).

## Technique #4. Feudal Lord Lifts the Tripod (Ba Wang Tai Ding, 霸王抬鼎)

Use ba wang tai ding when your opponent presses your chest with both of his hands.

Situation: Your opponent presses your chest with both of his hands.

Immediately turn your body to your right to neutralize the press, and grab his right wrist with your right hand while pushing his elbow to his left with your left hand.

Finally, reposition yourself and use the leverage generated from both of your hands to lock his right arm.

**Theory**

Misplacing the bone (elbow): Your right hand's grabbing is a pluck (cai, 採). To prevent him from turning his body, you should push the left side of your body against his right shoulder area.

### Technique #5. Arm Wraps Around the Dragon's Neck (Bi Chan Long Jing, 臂纏龍頸)

Use *bi chan long jing* when your opponent presses your chest with both of his hands.

Situation: Your opponent presses your chest with both of his hands.

Immediately reposition yourself to his right side, and raise your right forearm to lock his right forearm while pushing his elbow to his left with your left forearm.

Next, lock his right arm in front of your chest while placing your left arm on his throat.

Finally, circle your left arm around his neck to lock him.

## Theory

Misplacing the bone (elbow) and sealing the breath (neck): Your right hand's grabbing or locking is a pluck (cai, 採), your left arm's opening on his throat is a rend (lie, 挒), and finally, the arm wrapping around his neck is a coil (chan, 纏). To make this technique effective, you should keep his right arm bent and lock it in front of your chest.

## 3-5. Qin Na in An

*An* means to "stamp" or to "press down, forward, or upward" by the hand or hands. Offensively, *an* is normally used to strike a cavity in the chest area or to push the opponent off balance. Defensively, *an* is used to seal your opponent's wrists, arms, elbows, or even shoulder to immobilize the free movement of his upper limbs.

*An* used to strike the chest.

*An* used to push.

*An* used defensively to immobilize.

## I. Qin Na for An

Strictly speaking, the purpose of *an* is to strike or to seal. Therefore, there are not too many qin na techniques that can be ascribed to *an*. Here we can introduce only a few possible qin na for *an*.

## Technique #1. Feudal Lord Pushes the Cauldron (Ba Wang Tui Ding, 霸王推鼎)

Use ba wang tui ding when your opponent presses your right forearm with both of his hands.

Situation: Your opponent presses your right forearm with both of his hands.

Immediately step your left leg behind his right leg and turn your body to your right to neutralize the press. Coil your left hand around his right arm until it reaches his sacrum while placing your right hand on his chin.

Next, use the leverage created by your right hand and left hand to push his upper body backward to lock his spine.

If necessary, you may continue pushing until he falls.

**Theory**

Misplacing the bone (spine): When you circle your left hand around his right arm and reach his sacrum, it is a coil (chan, 纏). The final push from your right hand to his chin or upper body is a press down (an, 按). Your positioning is very important. A proper position offers you good leverage for pushing and safe distance from his left hand.

### Technique #2. Force the Bow (Qiang Po Ju Gong, 強迫鞠躬)

Use *qiang po ju gong* when both of your opponent's hands are pressing your right forearm.

Situation: Both of your opponent's hands are pressing your right forearm.

Immediately turn your body to your right, and step your left leg behind his right leg while grabbing his right wrist with your right hand.

Next, insert your left hand under his left armpit and reach the upper back of his head.

Finally, release your right hand and move it under his right armpit to reach the upper back of his head and press his head down with both hands to lock his neck. To avoid his kicking you, you should stand with one leg forward against his tailbone.

## Theory

Misplacing the bone (neck) and sealing the breath (windpipe): Your right hand's grabbing is a pluck (cai, 採) and both of your hands' pressing against the rear of his head is a press down (an, 按). To prevent him from straightening his arm and slipping down, you must press both of your hands on his upper head instead of his neck.

### Technique #3. Repulse the Monkey (Dao Nian Hou, 倒撵猴)

Use *dao nian hou* when both of your opponent's hands are pressing on your right forearm.

Situation: Both of your opponent's hands are pressing on your right forearm. Immediately turn your body to your right to neutralize his pushing or pressing while using your left hand to grab his right wrist.

Next, twist his left wrist counterclockwise while placing your right hand on his chin.

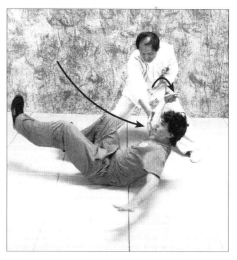

Then use the leverage generated from both of your hands to lock his left arm and head.

To take him down, you may simply increase your twisting and pushing pressure while circling him to your left.

Alternatively, once you have locked his wrist and head, you may step your right leg behind his right leg.

Then sweep your right leg backward to take him down.

## Theory

Dividing the muscle/tendon (wrist) and misplacing the bone (neck): Your left hand's grabbing is a pluck (cai, 採), and your right hand's forward pushing is a forward press (*an*, 按). This technique is not too effective if you wish to lock him in place. The locking is only to put him into an awkward position for your takedown.

**Technique #4. Double Hands Push the Mountain (Shuang Shou Tui Shan, 雙手推山)**

Use *shuang shou tui shan* when both of your opponent's hands are on your shoulders.

Situation: Both of your opponent's hands are on your shoulders. Immediately raise both of your arms up to the center.

Next, coil both of your hands around both his arms until they reach his upper chest.

Finally, push both of your hands forward and upward to his upper chest.

This will allow you to lock both his arms in front of your chest. You should beware of his knee striking you. If you lock him properly, he will not be able to kick you.

## Theory

Pressing the tendon (post-arm) and misplacing the bone (shoulder): When you raise both of your arms upward, it is an upward wardoff (peng, 掤), and when you circle your hands around his arms until they reach the upper chest, it is a coil (chan, 纏). Finally, the forward and upward pushing by both of your hands to his upper chest is an upward pushing (an, 按). This technique is useful only if both of your opponent's hands are grabbing you tightly. If he releases his grabbing while you are coiling your hands, you will not be able to lock his arm.

## II. Qin Na against An

Because the hand is open when *an* is applied, almost all of the qin na techniques against open hands can be used against *an*. Truly speaking, there are more than twenty qin na techniques that can be used against the open hand. Here we will introduce only some of them for your reference. If you are interested in learning more qin na against open hands, you should refer to *Comprehensive Applications of Shaolin Chin Na*, published by YMAA.

### Technique #1. White Crane Twists Its Neck (Bai He Niu Jing, 白鶴扭頸)

The bai he niu jing technique is used against your opponent when he is pressing or pushing your chest.

Situation: You discover your opponent's hand or hands are pressing or pushing toward your chest.

Immediately reposition yourself to his right side to avoid his pressing, while using your right hand to grab his right fingers and placing your left hand on his elbow.

Next, twist his fingers clockwise while pressing your left hand on his elbow to generate leverage for locking the base of his pinkie's tendons.

Under this lock, your opponent will have to follow your will. Therefore, you may circle him down to the ground for better control.

## Theory

Dividing the muscle/tendon (base of pinkie's tendon): Your right hand's grabbing is a pluck (cai, 採), and the final position of locking from both of your hands is a squeeze (ji, 擠). When you control your opponent, you should pay more attention to the base of his pinkie. Only when your mind is there are you able to lock his tendons effectively. Your left hand is only to offer you good leverage for your control.

## Technique #2. White Crane Covers Its Wings (Bai He Yan Chi, 白鶴掩翅)

The *bai he yan chi* technique is used against your opponent when he is pressing or pushing your chest.

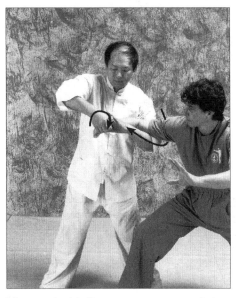

Situation: Your opponent uses his hand to push or press you. Immediately reposition yourself to his right while using your right hand to grab the fingers of his right hand and placing your left hand on his right elbow.

Next, twist his fingers to generate pain in the base of his pinkie, and move your left hand under his right arm and reach his pinkie.

Finally, use your left elbow to stop his right elbow from going down, while using your left middle finger to push the top of your right thumb to increase the twisting pressure on his pinkie's base tendons. This will allow you to lock his pinkie effectively.

## Theory

Dividing the muscle/tendon (base of pinkie's tendon): Your right hand's grabbing is a pluck (cai, 採), the final position of your right hand's twisting is a turning (zhuan, 轉), and your left middle finger's downward pressing is a downward press (*an*, 按). Again, when you control your opponent, you should pay more attention to the base of his pinkie. Only when your mind is there are you able to lock his tendons effectively. Your left hand is only to offer you good leverage for your control.

### Technique #3. White Crane Bores the Bush (Bai He Chuan Cong, 白鶴穿叢)

Bai he chuan cong is used against your opponent when he is pressing or pushing your chest.

Situation: Your opponent uses his right hand to press or push your chest. Use your right hand to grab the fingers of his right hand while placing your left hand on his right elbow.

Reposition yourself to his right side. Next, step your right leg behind his right leg while twisting his pinkie's tendons with your right hand and rotating his arm downward with the help of your left hand.

Finally, lock his right arm behind him while pushing his head to his left with your left hand, or simply pull his hair backward.

## Theory

Dividing the muscle/tendon (tendon on the base of the pinkie) and misplacing the bone (neck): Your right hand's grabbing is a pluck (cai, 採), the final locking position of your right hand and chest is a squeeze (ji, 擠), and your left hand's pushing against his head is a rend (lie, 挒). Once you have locked your opponent's arm behind him, and in order to increase the pain for your control, you should increase the pressure in twisting his pinkie's tendons.

**Technique #4. Butterfly Bores Through the Flowers (Hu Die Chuan Hua, 蝴蝶穿花)**

The *hu die chuan hua* technique is used against your opponent when his hand is approaching you.

Situation: Your opponent uses his right hand to press or push your chest. Reposition yourself to his right while also using your left hand to grab the fingers of his right hand from the back of his hand.

Next, circle his hand downward while using your right hand to lock his post-arm to prevent him from stepping and freeing himself.

Then step your right leg behind your left leg while circling his right arm behind him.

Finally, step your left leg behind him, twist his wrist counterclockwise, and push his chin to his left with your right hand.

## Theory

Dividing the muscle/tendon (wrist) and misplacing the bone (wrist and shoulder): Your left hand's grabbing is a pluck (cai, 採), and the final twisting of his wrist is a turning (zhuan, 轉). To make this technique most effective, you should twist his wrist strongly toward the rear side of his palm. This can generate great pain.

### Technique #5. The Child Worships the Buddha (Tong Zi Bai Fo, 童子拜佛)

The *tong zi bai fo* technique is used against the *an* force that has already reached your chest.

Situation: Your opponent has placed his hand on your upper chest and is ready to emit his pressing or pushing power. Immediately reposition yourself to yield to his pushing while grabbing the fingers of his right hand.

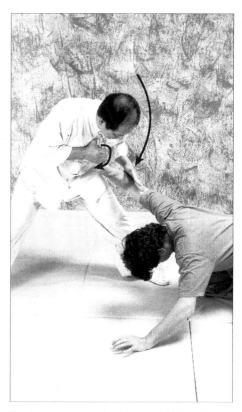

When you do this, you should also place your left hand on his right elbow to immobilize his elbow's movement. Next, turn his wrist ninety degrees clockwise with your right hand and lock it there.

Finally, bow your body toward him while using your left hand to keep his arm bent, and keep it lower than his wrist. This will offer you a great angle for locking.

## Theory

Dividing the muscle/tendon (wrist): Your right hand's grabbing is a pluck (cai, 採), the twisting of his wrist is a turning (zhuan, 轉), and the left hand's pushing downward against his elbow is a downward press (an, 按). To make this technique most effective, you should keep his elbow lower than his wrist. Naturally, the locking of his wrist from your right hand must be strong.

### Technique #6. Small Wrap Hand (Xiao Chan Shou, 小纏手)

The *xiao chan shou* technique is used against the situation in which your opponent's hands are already on your forearm to seal it downward.

Situation: Your opponent's hands are already on your forearm to seal it downward.

Immediately reposition yourself to his right while at the same time locking his fingers with your left hand and coiling your right hand on his wrist.

Finally, circle your wrist down to lock his wrist until his body reaches the ground.

## Theory

Dividing the muscle/tendon (wrist): When you move your right hand to the top of his wrist, it is a coil (chan, 纏), and the final downward pressing is a downward press (*an*, 按). In order to prevent him from escaping right from the beginning, you should use your fingers to push his index finger toward his wrist and cover all his other fingers tightly onto your forearm. When you press him down, a circular motion can generate a great locking pressure in his wrist.

### Technique #7. Upward Finger Turn (Shang Fen Zhi, 上分指)

Use *shang fen zhi* when both of your opponent's hands are on your right arm and are pressing it.

Situation: Both of your opponent's hands are on your right arm and are pressing it. Immediately place your left hand on his right hand.

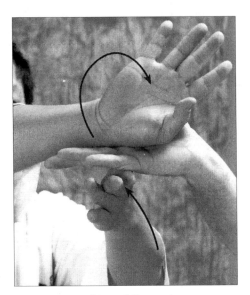

Next, reposition yourself to his right to neutralize his pressing or pushing while turning your right arm.

Finally, use your thumb and index finger to lock his index finger upward.

### Theory

Misplacing the bone (base of index finger): Your left hand's finger locking is a pluck (cai, 採). When you control him to the final position, your index finger should be on the base of his index finger with the support of the other three fingers, while the thumb is on the last joint of his index finger. If you can, you should keep his arm straight to have better control.

Keep the opponent's arm straight for better control.

### Technique #8. Large Rollback (Da Lu, 大擺)

Use da lu when both of your opponent's hands are on your right forearm.

Situation: Both of your opponent's hands are on your right forearm.

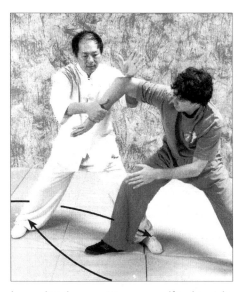

Immediately reposition yourself to his right while using your right hand to hook down and grab his right wrist and using your left forearm to press his elbow upward.

Then step your right leg backward. The leverage is generated from both of your hands to lead him down to the ground. Your left forearm should press on the rear post-arm tendon located about three inches above his elbow.

## Theory

Pressing the tendon (post-arm) and misplacing the bone (elbow): Your right hand's hooking and grabbing is a pluck (cai, 採). In fact, this entire action is large rollback (da lu, 大攦).

Press forward or press downward; *an* (按) is the most common technique in taiji pushing hands. Therefore, in order to become a proficient taiji martial artist, you should master those qin na techniques that can be used against *an*. As mentioned earlier, there are many techniques that can be used against open hands, such as *an* in taijiquan. We have introduced only some of the techniques. If you wish to know more about this, you should refer to *Comprehensive Applications of Shaolin Chin Na*, published by YMAA.

# Chapter 4: Qin Na in Cai, Lie, Zhou, and Kao

### 4-1. Introduction

As mentioned in the second chapter, cai, lie, zhou, and kao occupy the four corners in the taiji eight trigrams. This implies that, theoretically speaking, these four jing patterns are applied to the corners. However, you should not be strictly limited by these rules. When you apply the techniques, they are all alive and vary according to actual situations. In this chapter, we will introduce those qin na techniques that can be used from these four jing patterns, and also those that can be used against them.

### 4-2. Qin Na in Cai

Generally, pluck (cai, 採) is done by grabbing or locking part of your opponent's body and then either controlling it immediately, or leading the plucking downward or to the corners for some specific purposes—for example, to make him lose balance or to put him into an awkward situation. The part of the body plucked can be the finger, wrist, forearm, elbow, sleeves, clothes, or even the hair. The corners that the cai leads can be to the backward right, to the forward right, to the backward left, or to the forward left.

Cai used to lead the opponent backward right.

Cai used to lead the opponent forward right.

Cai used to lead the opponent backward left.

Cai used to lead the opponent forward left.

## I. Qin Na for Cai

You should remember that in taijiquan, cai, like the other seven jing patterns, is only *an* action that can be used to lock the opponent directly or is followed by pulling the opponent at an angle that can expose his cavities or vital areas for striking, or make him lose stability. Here we will introduce some of the qin na techniques that are related to the cai action.

Situation: Both of your opponent's hands are pressing your right forearm. Immediately turn your body to your right to neutralize his pressing.

### Technique #1. Left Right Cross Elbow (Zuo You Jiao Zhou, 左右交肘)

Use zuo you jiao zhou when both of your opponent's hands are pressing your right forearm.

At the same time, hook down and grab his right wrist, and place your left hand on his right elbow to control his arm.

In this situation, it is common that your opponent will punch to your face with his left fist. If this happens, immediately raise your left forearm to intercept his left-hand punch.

Finally, twist both of his arms and use his right arm to lock his left arm.

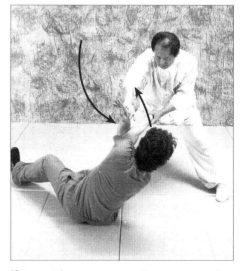

If you wish, you may continue your turning until he falls.

### Theory

Misplacing the bone (elbow) or pressing the tendon (post-arm): Your two-hand grabbing is a pluck (cai, 採), and the rotation of both arms is turning (zhuan, 轉). In order to make the technique effective, your opponent's left arm must be straight. The pressure generated from his right arm to his left arm should be either directly on the rear side of his elbow or on the tendons located about three inches above his elbow.

### Technique #2. White Crane Twists Its Neck (Bai He Niu Jing, 白鶴扭頸)

Use bai he niu jing if your opponent is in front of you with his right hand open.

Situation: Your opponent is in front of you with his right hand open.

Immediately reposition yourself to his right while grabbing his fingers with your right hand, and twist them toward his pinkie to lock his pinkie's base tendons.

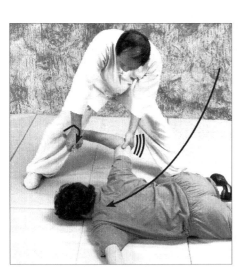

When you do this, you should also place your left hand on his right elbow and press it toward his right pinkie. This will offer you good leverage for locking. Finally, lead him down to the ground.

### Theory

Dividing the muscle/tendon (base of pinkie): Your right hand's grabbing is a pluck (cai, 採), and your left hand's pressing on his elbow is a squeeze (ji, 擠). The angle of locking his pinkie's tendon is very important. You should place your mind on this area while you are locking him.

### Technique #3. One Post to Support the Heavens (Yi Zhu Ding Tian, 一柱頂天)

Use *yi zhu ding tian* when your opponent's right hand is on your right forearm.

Situation: Your opponent's right hand is on your right forearm.

Immediately step your left leg to the front of his right leg while leading his arm to your right with your right hand and left elbow.

### Theory

Misplacing the bone (shoulder and elbow): Your two-hand grabbing is a pluck (cai, 採), and your left shoulder's upward supporting is an upward pressing (kao, 靠). The trick to using this technique correctly is to keep his entire arm straight and then lift it upward against his shoulder.

Finally, grab his hand with both of your hands, place your left shoulder under his right armpit, straighten out his entire arm, and then lift it upward to lock him. Your positioning is very important. The range should be beyond your opponent's left hand strike.

**Technique #4. Lead the Snake to Enter the Cave (Yin She Ru Dong, 引蛇入洞)**

Use yin she ru dong when both of your opponent's hands are pressing your right forearm.

Situation: Both of your opponent's hands are pressing your right forearm.

Immediately raise your right arm to neutralize his pushing or pressing, while using your left hand to grab his left wrist.

Next, lead his left arm down by locking his left elbow with both of your hands.

Finally, continue your locking until he is on the ground.

**Theory**

Misplacing the bone (elbow): When you raise your right forearm to neutralize his pressing, it is an upward wardoff (peng, 掤). Your left hand's wrist and right hand's elbow grabbing is a pluck (cai, 採). To make this technique effective, you must keep his arm straight. The pressure should be directly on the rear side of his elbow.

### Technique #5. Hands Grab Double Cavities (Shou Kou Shuang Xue, 手扣雙穴)

The *shou kou shuang xue* technique is a typical example of using the pluck (cai, 採) to grab a cavity.

Situation: Both of your opponent's hands are pressing your right forearm.

Immediately neutralize his pressing to your right. Grab his right wrist with your right hand while placing your left hand on his elbow.

Quchi
(Li-11)

Shaohai
(H-3)

Finally, bend his wrist with your right hand while grabbing the two cavities shaohai (H-3) and quchi (LI-11) with your left hand.

You should lock him upward so that he cannot kick you or punch you with his left hand.

## Theory

Dividing the muscle/tendon (wrist) and cavity press (shaohai and quchi cavities): Your right hand's grabbing on your opponent's wrist and your left hand's locking on his cavities are pluck (cai, 採). Occasionally, you will encounter an opponent whose cavities are not as sensitive as others'. In this case, this technique will not be effective. If you discover this, immediately use your right leg to kick his groin.

## II. Qin Na against Cai

Since cai is often used in actual taiji combat, there are many qin na techniques that have been developed against the plucking and grabbing. Here we will only introduce some of the typical qin na useful against cai. If you are interested in knowing more about qin na techniques against cai, you may refer to the book *Comprehensive Applications of Shaolin Chin Na*, published by YMAA.

### Technique #1. Small Wrap Hand (Xiao Chan Shou, 小纏手)

Use *xiao chan shou* when your opponent's right hand grabs your right wrist and his left hand grabs your elbow.

Situation: Your opponent's right hand grabs your right wrist and his left hand grabs your elbow.

Immediately reposition yourself to his right side, using your left hand to pull his index finger toward your wrist while raising your right arm to set up an advantageous angle to counter his grabbing.

Then wrap your right hand around the top side of his wrist to lock it.

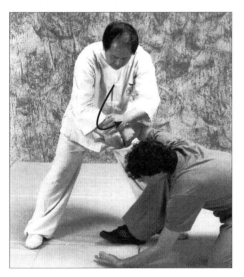

Finally, circle it downward to lock him.

### Theory

Dividing the muscle/tendon (wrist): Your two-hand wrapping is coil (chan, 纏), and the final pressing by your right hand is press down (*an*, 按). In order to lock your opponent efficiently, you must use your right fingers to direct his elbow and keep it slightly lower than his wrist. This will allow you to set up the best controlling angle on his wrist. When you apply this technique, the movement should be round and smooth. Only then are you able to control your opponent naturally, without alerting him to your intention.

**Technique #2. Large Wrap Hand (Da Chan Shou, 大纏手)**

Although *da chan shou* is very similar to small wrap hand (xiao chan shou), the method of achieving the final control is different.

Situation: Your opponent's right hand is grabbing your wrist while his left hand is controlling your right elbow.

Reposition yourself to his right side, and raise your right arm while moving your left hand under his forearm until it reaches his right hand.

Next, use your left hand to push his index finger toward your wrist while wrapping your right hand over his wrist.

Finally, bend your body toward him and press your right hand toward his wrist to lock him down to the ground.

Alternative application: Reposition yourself to his right side.

Move your left hand over your right palm and pull his or middle finger toward your wrist.

Then wrap your right hand around his wrist.

## Theory

Dividing the muscle/tendon (wrist): Your right hand's grabbing on his wrist and your left hand's locking on his cavities are pluck (cai, 採). Your two-hand wrapping is coil (chan, 纏), and the final pressing by your right hand is press down (an, 按). In order to lock him efficiently, you must use your right fingers to direct your opponent's elbow and keep it slightly lower than his wrist. This will allow you to set up the best controlling angle on his wrist.

Finally, using the leverage of both of your hands, bow toward him and lock him to the ground.

## Technique #3. Large Rollback (Da Lu, 大捋)

Use da lu if your opponent's right hand is grabbing your right wrist while his left hand is controlling your right elbow.

Situation: Your opponent's right hand is grabbing your right wrist while his left hand is controlling your right elbow.

Immediately reposition yourself to his right side while raising your right arm and placing your left forearm on the tendons of the rear of his post-arm.

Finally, step your right leg backward and use the leverage generated from both of your hands to lead him down to the ground.

### Theory

Pressing tendons (post-arm) and misplacing the bone (elbow): Your right hand's grabbing is a pluck (cai, 採), and your left forearm's rolling-back motion is a rollback (lu, 捋). In fact, this action is considered large rollback (da lu, 大捋) in taijiquan techniques. In order to make this technique effective, you must press his rear post-arm tendons on the right spot. The accurate position for pressing is about three inches above the elbow on the rear side of his post-arm. Naturally, you may also press his rear elbow to lock his elbow joint.

**Technique #4. Reverse Wrist Press / Crane Spreads Its Wings (Fan Ya Wan / Bai He Liang Chi, 反壓腕 / 白鶴亮翅)**

Use fan ya wan / bai he liang chi if your opponent's right hand is grabbing your right wrist while his left hand is controlling your right elbow.

Situation: Your opponent's right hand is grabbing your right wrist while his left hand is controlling your right elbow.

Immediately use your left hand to grab his right hand and try to free your right hand.

Next, use both of your hands to rotate his right wrist counterclockwise.

Finally, step your right leg behind his right leg, use your left hand to twist his right wrist continuously, and use your right forearm to push the upper back of his head forward.

## Theory

Dividing the muscle/tendon (wrist) and misplacing the bone (elbow, shoulder, and neck): Your left hand's grabbing is a pluck (cai, 採), your right hand's circling to free itself is a coil (chan, 纏), and finally, the forearm's pushing is a rend (lie, 挒). To make this technique effective, your opponent's right arm should not be bent too much nor kept too straight. A correct setup for the angle between the forearm and post-arm can make a significant difference in this technique.

## Technique #5. Hand Bends the Pine Branch (Shou Ban Song Zhi, 手扳松枝)

Use *shou ban song zhi* when your opponent's right hand is grabbing your right wrist while his left hand is controlling your right elbow.

Situation: Your opponent's right hand is grabbing your right wrist while his left hand is controlling your right elbow.

Immediately reposition yourself to his right side while rotating your right wrist counterclockwise to free yourself from his grabbing, and place your left hand on his index finger area.

Next, free your right wrist while using your left thumb and index finger to lock him.

### Theory

Misplacing the bone (base of index finger): Your final locking is a pluck (cai, 採). To make this technique most effective and to prevent your opponent from turning his body, you should keep his arm straight. The trick to keeping his arm straight is to lock his index finger while his arm is in a low position, and then lift his arm upward. In the final lock, the leverage generated from your thumb and index finger is the key to locking.

To make this technique most effective, you should place your thumb on the last joint of his index finger and your index finger on the base of his index finger.

## Technique #6. Old Man Promoted to General (Lao Han Bai Jiang, 老漢拜將)

Use *lao han bai jiang* when your opponent's right hand is grabbing your right wrist while his left hand is controlling your right elbow.

Situation: Your opponent's right hand is grabbing your right wrist while his left hand is controlling your right elbow.

Immediately step your left leg behind his right leg and cover his right hand with your left hand. Then circle your left elbow over his right arm and place the rear side of his right elbow under your left armpit.

Next, use the leverage of your hand's grabbing and your left armpit to lock him and lead him down to the ground.

When you lock his arm, you should also use both of your hands to control his right hand.

### Theory

Dividing the muscle/tendon (wrist) and misplacing the bone (elbow): Your two-hand grabbing is a pluck (cai, 採), and in the final lock, your shoulder's (armpit's) downward pressing is a press against (kao, 靠). To make this technique effective, you must keep your opponent's arm straight. If necessary, you may jerk your power and break his elbow easily.

## Technique #7. Wild Chicken Breaks Its Wings (Ye Ji Yao Chi, 野雞拗翅)

Use ye ji yao chi when your opponent's right hand is plucking or pressing your right shoulder.

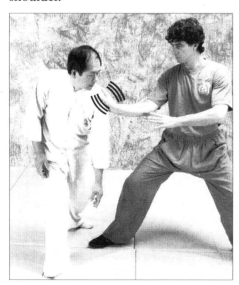

Situation: Your opponent's right hand is plucking or pressing your right shoulder.

Immediately use your right hand to grab his right hand while circling your left arm to the top of his right elbow.

Finally, reposition yourself to his right side while using the leverage generated from your right hand and left elbow to press him down to the ground.

**Theory**

Dividing the muscle/tendon (wrist) and misplacing the bone (elbow): Your two-hand grabbing is a pluck (cai, 採), and in the final lock, your elbow's pressing is elbow (zhou, 肘). The shoulder is one of the few common places at which your opponent can pluck you. He can either grab your clothes on the shoulder area and then pull you down to destroy the mobility of your arm, or grab your shoulder tendon to lock your shoulder area. To make this technique effective, you should keep his elbow bent and lower than his wrist. The major pain is generated from his wrist, not from his elbow.

## 4-3. Qin Na in Lie

As discussed in chapter 2, lie is the action of using the arm to split or rend in order to put your opponent into a locking position or to make him fall. Very often it is considered a sideways peng. However, strictly speaking, peng's power is more horizontal, and that of lie is more diagonal. Lie action is normally used against the neck, shoulder, or post-arm. Here we will introduce some typical examples of lie as applied in qin na.

Lie used against the neck.

Lie used against the shoulder.

### I. Qin Na for Lie

In order to use the arm for lie in qin na, often you will need to use the other hand to pluck (cai, 採) or control (na, 拿) your opponent's wrist. If the angle of lie is applied accurately, it is very easy to lock your opponent or to make him fall.

Lie used against the post-arm.

### Technique #1. Arm Wraps Around the Dragon's Neck (Bi Chan Long Jing, 臂纏龍頸)

Use bi chan long jing when both of your opponent's hands are on your right forearm and are pressing it.

Situation: Both of your opponent's hands are on your right forearm and are pressing it.

Immediately reposition yourself to his right side, and grab his right wrist with your right hand while using your left hand to push his right elbow to bend it.

Next, pull his right arm against your chest while using your left arm to push his neck backward.

Finally, circle your left arm around his neck and lock him upward until his heels are off the ground.

## Theory

Sealing the breath (neck) and misplacing the bone (shoulder and elbow): Your right hand's grabbing is a pluck (cai, 採), your left arm's pushing against his neck is a rend (lie, 挒), and in the final lock the arm's circling is a wrap (chan, 纏). This technique is derived from one of the taiji postures, diagonal flying. This technique cannot only lock his neck to seal his breath, but if necessary, you can also take him down.

## Technique #2. Reverse Wrist Press (Fan Ya Wan, 反壓腕)

Use *fan ya wan* when your opponent's hands are on your right arm, pressing it or simply sticking with it.

Situation: Your opponent's hands are on your right arm, pressing it or simply sticking.

Immediately use your left hand to grab his right wrist and twist it counterclockwise.

Next, step your right leg behind his right leg while using both hands to twist his right wrist strongly.

Finally, continue to control his wrist with your left hand and lock his arm on your stomach area while using your right arm to push the upper back of his head forward to lock his arm.

## Theory

Dividing the muscle/tendon (wrist) and misplacing the bone (shoulder, elbow, and neck): Your left hand's grabbing is a pluck (cai, 採), and your right arm's pushing against his rear upper neck is a rend (lie, 捌). The angle of locking is very important. The locking leverage is generated from the left hand's twisting and your right hand's pushing. His arm should not be too straight in the final locking.

### Technique #3. White Crane Twists Its Neck (Bai He Niu Jing, 白鶴扭頸)

Use bai he niu jing if your opponent is right in front of you with his right hand open, or he is trying to use his right hand to grab your chest.

Situation: Your opponent is right in front of you with his right hand open, or he may be trying to use his right hand to grab your chest.

Immediately step your left leg behind his right leg while using your right hand to grab the fingers of his right hand, and twisting them to the right and then toward him to control the base tendons of his pinkie.

Next, continue to twist his fingers with your right hand while using your left hand to push his chin backward.

Finally, circle him down to the ground as you continue to lock his right arm while using your left hand to push his head to his left. This will generate the leverage to lock his fingers, arms, and neck.

### Theory

Dividing the muscle/tendon (wrist) and misplacing the bone (neck): Your right hand's grabbing is a pluck (cai, 採), and your left arm's pushing his neck and then circling it down is a rend (lie, 挒). When you control your opponent's right arm, his arm should be bent ninety degrees for better control. Furthermore, his elbow should be slightly lower than his wrist. This can be done by controlling his pinkie's tendons. Right from the beginning until the end, you should keep his arm locked.

## Technique #4. Wild Horses Shear the Mane / Wave Hands in Clouds (Ye Ma Fen Zong / Yun Shou, 野馬分鬃 / 雲手)

Use *ye ma fen zong / yun shou* when both of your opponent's hands are on your right forearm. Immediately move your left forearm under his right forearm.

Situation: Both of your opponent's hands are on your right forearm. Immediately move your left forearm under his right forearm.

Next, turn your body to your left to neutralize his pushing, and grab his right wrist with your left hand while placing your right forearm under his post-arm.

Finally, use the leverage generated from your left hand and right forearm to lock him upward. You should stay on his right side to keep away from his left hand's possible attack.

Alternative application: You may use your right forearm to lock the tendons on the rear side of his post-arm.

## Theory

Misplacing the bone (shoulder) and pressing the tendon (post-arm): Your left hand's grabbing is a pluck (cai, 採), and your right arm's pressing against his post-arm is a rend (lie, 挒). If you are locking the tendons in his post-arm, the location of your right forearm's pressing on his post-arm is very important. The correct position should be about three inches above the elbow on the rear side of his post-arm. Often these two qin na are only used to uproot or lock your opponent temporarily. After locking, you may then strike his groin with your right knee or even swing him down to the ground.

### Technique #5. Grasp Sparrow's Tail (Lan Qiu Wei, 攬雀尾)

Use *lan qiu wei* when both of your opponent's hands are on your right forearm.

Situation: Both of your opponent's hands are on your right forearm.

Immediately reposition yourself to his right side and grab his right wrist with your right hand while using your right hand to push his elbow upward to keep it straight.

Next, pull his right arm toward your right while placing your left shoulder under his armpit.

Finally, turn your body to your left slightly and pull his right arm down to lock it on your left shoulder.

## Theory

Misplacing the bone (elbow and shoulder): Your right hand's grabbing is a pluck (cai, 採), and your left arm's upward diagonal locking is a rend (lie, 挒). The other option of locking is to place the tendons on the rear side of his post-arm on your left shoulder and use your left shoulder to press his tendons while pulling his arm down with both of your hands.

## II. Qin Na against Lie

As mentioned earlier, lie is commonly done with two hands. When one hand is grabbing or plucking the opponent's wrist, the other arm is used to generate the rending or splitting force. If your opponent uses lie against you, you have two options in applying qin na. One is to take care of the hand that is grabbing or plucking your wrist, and the other is to control the arm that is rending you. Since you have already learned how to use qin na against pluck (cai, 採) in the last section, we will not repeat it here. Here we will focus on the qin na against the rending arm.

### Technique #1. Left Right Cross Elbow (Zuo You Jiao Zhou, 左右交肘)

Use zuo you jiao zhou when your opponent's right hand grabs your right wrist while his left arm is on your neck, pushing backward.

Situation: Your opponent's right hand grabs your right wrist while his left arm is on your neck, pushing backward.

Immediately use your left hand to intercept his left arm and grab his wrist while raising your right forearm to loosen his grabbing.

Next, grab his right wrist with your right hand and cross his arms in front of him.

Finally, rotate both of his arms counterclockwise and use his right forearm to lock his left arm.

If you wish, you may sweep your right leg backward to take him down.

## Theory

Misplacing the bone (elbow and shoulder): Your two-hand grabbing is a pluck (cai, 採), and the twisting of both of his arms is a turning (zhuan, 轉). In order to make the locking effective, you must keep his left arm straight. When you execute this technique, you must be fast. The reason for this is simply that your opponent will have the same opportunity to execute the same technique to lock your arms. The first one executing the technique will be the one who controls.

### Technique #2. Carry a Pole on the Shoulder (Jian Tiao Bian Dan, 肩挑扁擔)

Use *jian tiao bian dan* when your opponent's right hand grabs your right wrist while his left arm is pressing against your neck.

Situation: Your opponent's right hand grabs your right wrist while his left arm is pressing against your neck. Immediately use your left hand to grab his left wrist to prevent him from pressing your neck.

Next, turn your body to your left while placing the rear tendons of his post-arm or armpit on your right shoulder.

If his tendons are on your shoulder, you may simply pull his arm down to generate pain in his tendons. However, if his armpit is on your shoulder, then you should pull his arm downward and then push upward toward his shoulder to create pain in his shoulder's tendons and ligaments.

## Theory

Misplacing the bone (elbow and shoulder) and pressing the tendon (post-arm): Your left hand's grabbing is a pluck (cai, 採), and your shoulder's upward pushing is an upward press (kao, 靠). If you are locking his tendons, you should raise your stance. This will offer you better leverage for locking. However, if you are locking his shoulder, then the movement of pulling his arm down to keep it straight first and then pushing it upward against his shoulder is the key to locking.

**Technique #3. Old Man Carries the Fish on His Back (Lao Han Bei Yu, 老漢背魚)**

Use lao han bei yu when your opponent's left hand grabs your left wrist and his right arm is pushing your neck.

Situation: Your opponent's left hand grabs your left wrist and his right arm is pushing your neck. Immediately use your right hand to grab his right wrist.

Next, reposition yourself while bending his arm with your right hand and chin.

Finally, free your left hand and use both hands to pull his arm downward to lock him on your back.

## Theory

Misplacing the bone (elbow and shoulder): Your right hand's grabbing is a pluck (cai, 採), and the final lock behind you is a shoulder upward press (kao, 靠). Whenever your wrist is grabbed, you should try to free it as soon as possible. The trick to freeing the wrist is to dislodge it through the space between your opponent's thumb and index finger. When you lock your opponent's arm, it should not be either too straight or too bent. The correct angle can make the technique very easy and effective to execute.

**Technique #4. Two Children Worship the Buddha (Shuang Tong Bai Fo, 雙童拜佛)**

Use *shuang tong bai fo* when your opponent's left hand grabs your left wrist while his right arm is pushing your neck.

Situation: Your opponent's left hand grabs your left wrist while his right arm is pushing your neck. Immediately use your right hand to grab his right wrist and push it forward to prevent his locking.

Then bow your body downward while pulling his right arm backward and pressing your left shoulder forward.

## Theory

Misplacing the bone (elbow and shoulder): Your right hand's grabbing is a pluck (cai, 採), and your left shoulder's pressing is a downward press (kao, 靠). This technique can only lock your opponent temporarily. If you wish, you may sweep your left leg backward while swinging his body to your right to take him down.

## 4-4. Qin Na in Zhou

As explained in chapter 2, the purpose of zhou is to use the elbow to strike the cavity (da, 打), to press the body (ji, 擠), to neutralize the opponent's press or push (hua, 化), to wrap or coil the opponent's limbs (chan, 纏), or to seal the opponent's attack (feng, 封). In taijiquan, zhou has an important role in qin na applications. When zhou is used for qin na, normally it must be coordinated with plucking or grabbing (cai, 採) on the opponent's wrist. Only then can zhou qin na be effective and powerful.

## I. Qin Na for Zhou

When zhou is used for qin na, the actions of pressing, neutralizing, wrapping, coiling, and sealing are critical for making the techniques effective. Because of this, the sensitivity of feeling the angles that are pressed, neutralized, wrapped, and sealed is very important. That means the "listening jing" (*ting jing*) on the elbow is the key to locking. With a correct angle of locking, the techniques can be executed without too much effort. Here we will introduce some typical examples.

### Technique #1. Prop Up Elbow (Shang Jia Zhou, 上架肘)

Use shang jia zhou when both of your opponent's hands are on your right arm and are pushing it.

Situation: Both of your opponent's hands are on your right arm and are pushing it.

Immediately use your left hand to grab his right hand.

Next, step your right leg behind his right leg and twist his right wrist with your left hand while circling your right elbow to the outside of his right elbow.

Finally, use the leverage of your left hand and right elbow to lock his arm.

If you wish, you may continue to step your left leg behind him while using your right arm and chest area to lock his right arm, and using your left hand to push the upper back of his head forward.

## Theory

Misplacing the bone (elbow and neck) and dividing the muscle/tendon (wrist): Your left hand's grabbing is a pluck (cai, 採), your elbow's circling and upward pushing is an elbow (zhou, 肘), and the final lock using your left hand to push the upper back of his head forward is a wardoff (peng, 掤). When you circle your elbow to lock his elbow, your left hand's twisting of his right wrist is very important. In fact, in order to increase your locking power, you should use both of your hands to handle the job. In the final lock, the best way to generate good leverage for the locking is to raise your right arm's locking while pushing the top of his head forward.

Locking with both hands.

Locking by raising your right arm while pushing the top of the opponent's head forward.

### Technique #2. Forgive Me for Not Going with You (Shu Bu Tong Xing, 恕不同行)

Use *shu bu tong xing* when both of your opponent's hands are on your right forearm and are pushing on it.

Situation: Both of your opponent's hands are on your right forearm and are pushing it.

Immediately use your left hand to grab his left hand.

Next, circle your right elbow on the top of his left elbow while twisting his left wrist with your left hand.

Finally, use the leverage of your left hand and right elbow to lock his left arm.

## Theory

Misplacing the bone (elbow) and dividing the muscle/tendon (wrist): Your left hand's grabbing is a pluck (cai, 採), and your right elbow's circling and pressing is an elbow (zhou, 肘). When you use your elbow to press him down, his elbow should be bent and slightly lower than his wrist. Naturally, you should position yourself in the right spot, beyond his right hand's attack.

## Technique #3. Turn the Body to Seize the Monkey (Fan Shen Qin Yuan, 翻身擒猿)

Use *fan shen qin yuan* when your opponent is behind you and his left hand is on your right shoulder.

Situation: Your opponent is behind you and his left hand is on your right shoulder.

Immediately use your left hand to grab his left wrist while circling your elbow upward.

Next, circle your right arm under his left elbow and raise it upward while releasing your left hand's wrist grabbing.

Finally, extend your right arm and use your right hand to push his chest to generate pain in his entire left arm.

**Theory**

Misplacing the bone (elbow and shoulder): Your left hand's grabbing is a pluck (cai, 採), your right elbow's circling around his arm is an elbow (zhou, 肘), and the final position of the hand's pushing is a wardoff (peng, 掤). When you lock your opponent's arm, prevent him from rotating his arm. If he can do that, he will be able to escape.

### Technique #4. The Hero Shows Courtesy (Ying Xiong You Li, 英雄有禮)

Use *ying xiong you li* when your opponent's right hand is on your left shoulder.

Situation: Your opponent's right hand is on your left shoulder.

Immediately step your right leg backward, and grab his right hand with your right hand while placing your left elbow on his right elbow.

Finally, twist his right wrist with your right hand, and press his elbow down with your left elbow while bowing your body toward him.

**Theory**

Dividing the muscle/tendon (wrist): Your right hand's grabbing is a pluck (cai, 採), and left elbow's pressing is an elbow (zhou, 肘). The main locking is on his wrist by your right hand. Your elbow's pressing is to maintain a good angle for the wrist's locking. His elbow should be slightly lower than his wrist.

## Technique #5. Daoist Greets with Hands (Dao Zi Zuo Ji, 道子作揖)

Use *Dao zi zuo ji* when your opponent uses his right hand to grab your right wrist.

Situation: Your opponent uses his right hand to grab your right wrist. Immediately circle your right hand counterclockwise to free yourself from the grabbing while placing your left forearm on his right elbow.

Next, circle your right hand around his right forearm until your right forearm is on his right forearm.

Finally, press his forearm downward with your right forearm while using your left elbow to push his right elbow upward.

## Theory

Misplacing the bone (elbow and shoulder): In the final locking, your right wrist's downward pressing against his forearm is a downward press (*an*, 按), and your left elbow's lifting on his elbow is an elbow (zhou, 肘). When you execute this technique, you must be fast. Otherwise, your opponent will have a chance to escape if he feels your locking.

### Technique #6. Extending the Neck for Water (Yin Jing Qiu Shui, 引頸求水)

Use yin jing qiu shui whenever you have a chance to grab your opponent's right fingers with your right hand.

Situation: You have a chance to grab your opponent's right hand fingers with your right hand. Immediately press his elbow toward his left.

Next, coil your left hand around his right arm until it reaches his post-arm near the elbow and lift his arm upward to lock it.

Finally, use your right hand to either push his chin upward or push it toward his left. This will offer you good leverage to generate pain in his right shoulder.

**Theory**

Misplacing the bone (shoulder): Your right hand's grabbing is a pluck (cai, 採), your left hand's circling around his right arm is a coil (chan, 纏), the left elbow's upward lifting on his forearm is an elbow (zhou, 肘), and your right hand's lifting on his chin is a lift (ti, 提). To make this technique effective, you must keep his right arm bent. If he is able to straighten his arm, it will not be effective. The trick to doing this is to use your left post-arm to prevent him from straightening his arm.

### Technique #7. Forward Upward Turning (Qian Shang Fan, 前上翻)

Use qian shang fan when your opponent's right hand is on your left forearm.

Situation: Your opponent's right hand is on your left forearm.

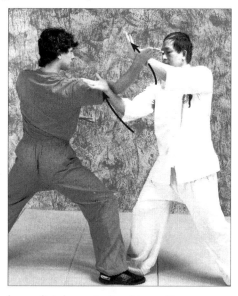

Immediately neutralize his pushing or grabbing to your left while using your right forearm to pull in his right elbow.

Next, step your right leg behind his right leg and use both hands to lock his arm backward.

Finally, let your right hand continue to lock his arm while using your left hand to push the upper back of his head forward to lock him.

## Theory

Misplacing the bone (elbow, shoulder, and neck): Your two-hand locking on his arm is a downward press (*an*, 按), and the final lock, which uses your elbow to lift up his elbow to lock his arm, is an elbow (*zhou*, 肘). The leverage generated from your right arm's locking and left hand's pushing on his head is the key to the locking. If you push his head too hard, you will pop his shoulder out of its socket.

The best method of locking his arm is to make the angle between his forearm and post-arm ninety degrees.

## II. Qin Na against Zhou

For emitting power (fa jing, 發勁) in taijiquan, the legs are the root of power, the waist is the steering wheel that controls the direction of the power's manifestation, and the hands are the places from which the power is manifested. The power can also be generated from the arm. For an arm, the shoulder is the root of the movement, the elbow is the steering wheel that controls the direction of the movement, and the hands are the final places where the movement ends. From this you can see that if you are able to immobilize your opponent's elbow movement, then you have restrained the free movements of his arms. Naturally, you will have governed the entire fighting situation.

For this reason, there were many qin na created in the past that can now be used to control the elbow. This is especially important when your opponent's hands are closed as fists, or when the fighting range is close. When your opponent's hands are closed, it is hard to control the fingers or even the wrist, and when the fighting range is close, the elbows and the shoulders will have become the main weapons for short-range fighting. Here we will introduce some qin na techniques that were specially designed against the elbow.

### Technique #1. Small Elbow Wrap (Xiao Chan Zhou, 小纏肘)

Use xiao chan zhou when your opponent uses his elbow to strike your solar plexus area.

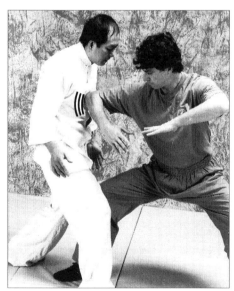

Situation: Your opponent uses his elbow to strike your solar plexus area.

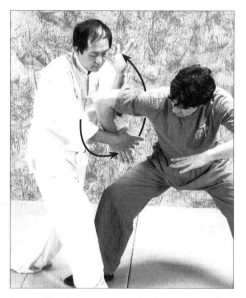

Immediately use your right forearm and your left arm to intercept and neutralize the attack.

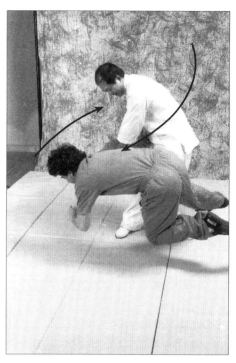

Next, reposition yourself, grab his right wrist with your right hand, and use the leverage created by both hands to rotate his arm and force him to bow.

Finally, step your right leg backward and circle him down to the ground.

## Theory

Misplacing the bone (elbow and shoulder): Your right hand's grabbing is a pluck (cai, 採), and the entire movement is a large rollback (da lu, 大擺). The pressure that makes your opponent follow your circle is generated from the leverage of both hands' controlling instead of pulling. Naturally, if you wish, you may also sweep your left leg backward to make him fall.

## Technique #2. Pressing Shoulder with a Single Finger or Extending the Neck for Water (Yi Zhi Ding Jian / Yin Jing Qiu Shui, 一指頂肩 / 引頸求水)

Use yi zhi ding jian / yin jing qiu shui when your opponent uses his elbow to strike your solar plexus.

Situation: Your opponent uses his elbow to strike your solar plexus. Use both arms to intercept and neutralize his attempt.

Next, reposition yourself, grab his right wrist with your right hand while coiling your left hand around his right arm until it reaches his post-arm near the elbow, and lock his right arm upward.

Finally, use your right index or middle finger to press his jianneiling (M-UE-48) cavity to create pain.

Alternative application: You may use your right hand to push his chin upward while lifting his right arm upward.

### Theory

Misplacing the bone (elbow and shoulder): Your right hand's grabbing is a pluck (cai, 採), your left hand's circling around his arm is a coil (chan, 纏), and your left arm and elbow's upward lifting to his right arm is elbow (zhou, 肘). The right index or middle finger's upward pressing to the jianneiling is a point (dian, 點), and finally, your right hand's upward lifting of his chin is a lift (ti, 提). Once you have locked his right arm behind him, the tendons and ligaments in his shoulder should be very tensed. In this case, if you press his jianneiling (M-UE-48, 肩內陵) cavity, significant pain can be produced. This is an example of using elbow (zhou, 肘) against elbow (zhou, 肘).

### Technique #3. Daoist Greets with Hands / Old Man Carries the Fish on His Back (Dao Zi Zuo Ji / Lao Han Bei Yu, 道子作揖 / 老漢背魚)

Use *Dao zi zuo ji / lao han bei yu* when your opponent uses his elbow to attack your solar plexus.

Situation: Your opponent uses his elbow to attack your solar plexus. Immediately use your left forearm to push his elbow downward to neutralize it.

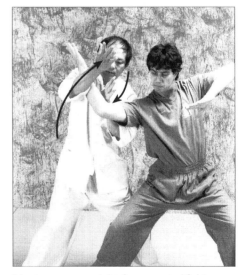

Next, use your right forearm to lift his right forearm while pushing his right elbow to his left with your left elbow.

Finally, rotate his arm until it is locked.

Alternative application: You may continue your turning and use your upper back to support the locking of his arm behind your back.

Locking angle should be neither too straight nor too bent.

## Theory

Misplacing the bone (elbow and shoulder): Your left forearm's pressing against his elbow strike is a downward press (*an*, 按), and in the final position, your left elbow's upward lifting is an elbow (*zhou*, 肘), while your right hand's downward pushing is a downward press (*an*, 按). This is another example of using the elbow (*zhou*, 肘) against the elbow (*zhou*, 肘). In the final locking, in order to prevent your opponent from turning around, you may use your left shoulder to push against his shoulder. In this case, your left shoulder's push is a press against (*kao*, 靠). In the optional technique, the support from your back for the locking is a press against (*kao*, 靠). The locking angle of his arm is very important. His arm should be neither too straight nor too bent.

## 4-5. Qin Na in Kao

As explained in chapter 2, the purpose of kao is to use part of your body to bump your opponent's body to make him lose his balance or fall. When your opponent is in the situation of regaining his balance, take this opportunity to execute further action such as kicking or striking. The common kao are done by the shoulder (jian kao, [shoulder kao], 肩靠), back (bei kao, [back kao], 背靠), hip (tun kao, [hip kao], 臀靠), thigh (tui kao, [leg kao], 腿靠), knee (xi kao, [knee kao], 膝靠), and chest (xiong kao, [chest kao], 胸靠). In addition, from the direction of kao, it can be distinguished as forward kao (qian kao, 前靠), downward kao (xia kao, 下靠), sideward kao (ce kao, 側靠), and upward kao (shang kao, 上靠).

### I. Qin Na for Kao

Though there are many types of kao, there are only a few that can be used for qin na. Often, kao is used to bump the opponent off his balance instead of locking or controlling. Here a few examples are introduced from which the kao can be used for qin na.

### Technique #1. Two Children Worship the Buddha (Shuang Tong Bai Fo, 雙童拜佛)

Use shuang tong bai fo when your opponent locks your right arm with both of his hands.

Situation: Your opponent locks your right arm using both of his hands to set up for lie (rend).

Immediately reposition yourself to his right side, and spin your right arm counterclockwise to escape from his locking while placing your left arm under his right armpit.

Next, bow your body forward, pulling his right forearm backward while pushing your left shoulder against his right shoulder, and lock him there.

**Theory**

Misplacing the bone (shoulder and elbow): In the final locking, your chest's forward pushing against his arm is a chest press against (xiong kao, 胸靠), while your left shoulder's pressing against his shoulder is a shoulder press against (jian kao, 肩靠). This technique can be used to control your opponent only temporarily. In fact, it can be used to swing him down to the ground.

## Technique #2. Old Man Promoted to General (Lao Han Bai Jiang, 老漢拜將)

Use lao han bai jiang when both of your opponent's hands are on your right arm and are pressing.

Situation: Both of your opponent's hands are pressing on your right arm.

Immediately use your left hand to grab his left hand while circling your right arm upward.

Next, turn your body to your left and place your right armpit on his left shoulder.

Finally, use the leverage generated from both of your hands' grabbing and your right shoulder to press him down to the ground.

### Theory

Misplacing the bone (shoulder and elbow): Your two-hand grabbing is a pluck (cai, 採), and the final lock is a shoulder press against (jian kao, 肩靠). To prevent his arm from bending, lock his elbow under your armpit. If necessary, you may use the jerking jing to break his elbow.

**Technique #3. Carry a Pole on the Shoulder (Jian Tiao Bian Dan, 肩挑扁擔)**

Use jian tiao bian dan when your opponent uses his right arm to rend your neck while grabbing your left wrist with his left hand.

Situation: Your opponent uses his right arm to generate lie (rend) force on your neck while grabbing your left wrist with his left hand. Immediately grab his right wrist with your right hand.

Next, turn your body to your right and place his post-arm on your left shoulder.

Finally, pull his arm first downward, and then lift it upward against his shoulder to generate strain in his shoulder's tendons and ligaments. Naturally, you may use your left shoulder to press upward against his tendons on his post-arm.

## Theory

Misplacing the bone (shoulder and elbow) and pressing the tendon (post-arm): Your right hand's grabbing is a pluck (cai, 採), and your shoulder's upward pressing is an upward press against (kao, 靠). If you are locking his shoulder, to make the technique effective, first, you pull his arm downward to straighten it out, and then push straight upward against his shoulder. This motion can generate great pain in his shoulder.

**Technique #4. Old Man Carries the Fish on His Back (Lao Han Bei Yu, 老漢背魚)**

Use lao han bei yu when your opponent uses his left hand to grab your left wrist while using his right arm to lie (rend) your neck.

Situation: Your opponent uses his left hand to grab your left wrist while using his right arm to rend your neck. Immediately use your right hand to grab his right wrist to prevent his rend.

Next, turn your body to your right and bend his arm while trying to free your left hand.

Finally, bow forward and use both of your hands to pull his arm down to lock him behind your back.

## Theory

Misplacing the bone (shoulder and elbow): Your right hand's grabbing is a pluck (cai, 採), and in the final position, your back's upward press is a press against (kao, 靠). When you control his arm, to make this technique effective, his arm should be neither too bent nor too straight.

### Technique #5. The Knee Presses the Enemy's Leg (Xi Ding Di Tui, 膝頂敵腿)

This technique, *xi ding di tui*, uses the knee to press against the opponent's leg or knee.

Situation: The distance between you and your opponent is short. Immediately hook your right leg behind his right leg.

Next, use the leg near the knee to press against the internal side of his calf to lock his right leg.

The angle of pressing is the key to the locking. With correct locking, you may lock his leg or even force him down easily.

### Theory

Misplacing the bone (knee): This action is a knee press against (xi kao, 膝靠). In a battle, this technique can be used very quickly, which allows you to put your opponent in a locked position temporarily or to make him fall. This technique is not designed to lock his leg permanently.

**Technique #6. The Leg Twists the Enemy's Leg (Tui Ban Di Tui, 腿絆敵腿)**

This technique *tui ban di tui* is very similar to xi ding di tui. The only difference is that you are locking from the external side of his leg.

Situation. The distance between you and your opponent is short. You may immediately use your left foot to hook his right leg near the ankle.

Then use the upper part of your calf or knee to press him.

## Theory

Misplacing the bone (knee): This action is a knee press against (xi kao, 膝靠). In a battle, this technique can be used very quickly, which allows you to put your opponent in a locked position temporarily or make him fall. This technique is not designed to lock his leg permanently.

## II. Qin Na against Kao

Most qin na techniques against kao focus on the shoulder kao. The reason for this is that when your opponent uses his shoulder to press against (kao, 靠), then you may have a chance to control his arms. If he uses another portion of the body, such as his chest, back, thigh, or knee, then it is very hard to execute any qin na technique against him. In this section, we will introduce some of the techniques useful against shoulder kao.

## Technique #1. Large Rollback (Da Lu, 大捋)

Use da lu when your opponent uses his right shoulder or upper arm to strike you.

Situation: Your opponent uses his right shoulder or upper arm to strike you.

Immediately use your right hand to control his right forearm while placing your left forearm on the rear tendon of his right post-arm. Your left palm should face downward.

### Theory

Misplacing the bone (shoulder and elbow) and pressing the tendon (rear post-arm): This technique uses large rollback (da lu, 大捋) against the kao. Your right hand's controlling of his forearm is a pluck (cai, 採). If your opponent uses his shoulder or upper arm to strike you, the way to prevent his attacking power from reaching you is to control his post-arm. Therefore, this technique can be effectively used against this strike. Naturally, you should use the circular motion to destroy his balance while both of your arms are leading him down to the ground.

Next, step your right leg backward and use the leverage of your right hand and left forearm to press him down to the ground. When you press him down, you should press your left forearm hard on his rear post-arm tendon while rotating your left forearm counterclockwise until your left palm is facing you. This left forearm rotation action will generate great pain in your opponent's post-arm, and therefore he will follow you to the ground.

**Technique #2. Two Children Worship the Buddha (Shuang Tong Bai Fo, 雙童拜佛)**

Use shuang tong bai fo when your opponent is pressing against your chest with his shoulder.

Situation: Your opponent is pressing against your chest with his shoulder.

Immediately use your right hand to control his right forearm while inserting your left arm under his right arm and pressing against his stomach area.

**Theory**

Misplacing the bone (shoulder and elbow) and pressing the tendon (rear post-arm): This technique uses shoulder press against (kao, 靠) to counterattack the shoulder press against (kao, 靠). Naturally, your right hand's controlling is a pluck (cai, 採). This technique can only be used to lock your opponent temporarily for further attack, such as using your right hand to strike his face, or even to circle him down.

Then bow your body forward while using the leverage generated from your right hand's pulling and left shoulder's downward pressing to lock his right arm.

### Technique #3. Daoist Greets with Hands / Old Man Carries the Fish on His Back (Dao Zi Zuo Ji / Lao Han Bei Yu, 道子作揖 / 老漢背魚)

Use Dao zi zuo ji / lao han bei yu when your opponent uses his right shoulder to press against your chest.

Situation: Your opponent uses his right shoulder to press against your chest.

Next, use the leverage generated from both of your hands and left elbow to lock his arm.

Close up of lock.

Alternative application: You may continue your turning and use your upper back to support the locking of his arm behind your back.

## Theory

Misplacing the bone (elbow and shoulder): Your left forearm's pressing against his elbow strike is a downward press (*an*, 按), and in the final position, your left elbow's upward lifting is an elbow (zhou, 肘), while your right hand's downward pushing is a downward press (an, 按). In the final locking, in order to prevent your opponent from turning around, you may use your left shoulder to push against his shoulder. In this case, your left shoulder's push is a press against (kao, 靠). In the optional technique, the support from your back for the locking is a press against (kao, 靠). The locking angle of his arm is very important. His arm should be neither too straight nor too bent.

### Technique #4. Arm Wraps Around the Dragon's Neck (Bi Chan Long Jing, 臂纏龍頸)

Use bi chan long jing when your opponent is pressing against your chest with his right shoulder.

Situation: Your opponent is pressing against your chest with his right shoulder. Immediately control his right forearm with your right hand and press his elbow down with your left forearm.

Next, reposition yourself and pull his right arm backward against your chest while circling your left arm toward his neck.

Finally, lock his arm on your chest while wrapping his neck with your left arm.

## Theory

Misplacing the bone (shoulder and elbow) and seal the breath (neck): This technique uses rend (lie, 挒) to counterattack the shoulder press against (kao, 靠). Your right hand's controlling is a pluck (cai, 採), and your left arm's wrapping is a rend (lie, 挒) and coil (chan, 纏).

From the techniques discussed in chapter 3 and chapter 4, you should have realized and comprehended two important points. First, the same technique can be applied in different situations, even though the setup and execution of the technique can be different. Second, among the eight basic taiji technical movements, it is easy to use one against the other in qin na. This is not surprising, given that these eight basic patterns were created to mutually support and conquer each other. Third, almost all qin na techniques introduced here can be applied in taiji pushing hands. This is again not surprising. This is simply because all the taiji pushing hands techniques are built upon the common foundation of these eight basic moving technical patterns.

# Chapter 5: Qin Na Applications in Taijiquan Postures

## 5-1. Introduction

In the last two chapters we have discussed the possible qin na applications in the eight basic taiji moving patterns: peng, lu, ji, *an*, cai, lie, zhou, and kao. In addition, qin na that may be used against these eight basic moving actions have also been introduced. However, if you analyze the thirty-seven postures of taiji movement (Yang Style), you will realize that although most of the postures are derived from the same eight basic movements, many others do not carry the same patterns and theory.

In this chapter, we will try to find the possible and reasonable qin na applications for these other taiji postures. There are, however, a very few of these postures from which I cannot find reasonable qin na techniques, and thus they will not be discussed. Furthermore, because I am only familiar with Yang Style Taijiquan, I can only offer you the possible qin na in Yang Style. However, since the basic theories of qin na remain the same in every style, after you have reached a good level of understanding, you may apply these same theories in other styles. If you would like to know more about striking and wrestling (taking down) techniques in taijiquan, you may refer to *Tai Chi Chuan Martial Applications*, published by YMAA.

Other than introducing those qin na categorized as "dividing the muscle/tendon" and "misplacing the bone," we would also like to offer you some information about cavity pressing or cavity striking in this chapter.

The technique of cavity grabbing, pressing, or striking is known as one of the highest martial techniques in China. You should know that, strictly speaking, when a cavity is attacked by grabbing or pressing—or both—it is classified as qin na. However, if the cavity is attacked by striking or kicking, then it will be classified in the fighting categories of striking and kicking.

In ancient times, almost every Chinese martial style trained cavity pressing or striking techniques. However, usually the highest level of these techniques was taught only to the trusted students who had stayed with the master for more than ten years. There are two main reasons for this. First, the theory is very deep, and the training is much harder than other martial training. Therefore, it is very difficult for a beginner to learn and reach a high level. Second, when many of the cavities are struck, it can cause death easily. For this reason, unless a student's morality is very high, normally a master would prefer to keep these secrets to himself instead of passing them down to immoral students.

It is the same in taijiquan. Although it is well known in China that taijiquan specializes in cavity press techniques, not too many taiji practitioners today know about them or train them. The main reason for this is that training cavity press takes a great deal of time and patience. It is especially hard to train in today's lifestyle, when most people are busy earning money for surviving or spending most of their leisure time in pursuit of entertainment. In addition to this, there are not too many taiji masters today who still have the knowledge and capability for teaching this art. Furthermore, even after you have trained this art today, you will never have a chance to use it, since it can cause death so easily. This situation is not the same as in ancient times, when every martial technique was critical for survival. It was more frequent that you had the opportunity to verify the effectiveness of your techniques. Today, most taiji masters emphasize pushing hands and teach students how to destroy the opponent's root, center, and balance. Actual combat in taijiquan has lost its meaning.

In this chapter, though you will see some introduction to cavity grabbing or striking, it is not intended to teach you and make you become a proficient taiji cavity press expert. In the second section of this chapter, some common hand forms for cavity press in taijiquan will also be summarized. Finally, in the third section, those qin na applications and cavity attacks for the taijiquan postures will be discussed.

## 5-2. Hand Forms for Cavity Press

In this section, we will summarize some of the hand forms that are commonly used in taiji cavity press. Since we do not intend to discuss this subject at a profound level, we will not include how to condition the hand forms, the herbs required for training, and the most important parts of the cavity press—the detailed skills and timing of striking. The reason for this is simply that it would take another entire book to discuss these subjects.

## A. Hand forms of cavity grabbing

### 1. Crane claw

Crane claw. Cavity-grabbing hand form.

### 2. Eagle claw

Eagle claw. Cavity-grabbing hand form.

3. Double-finger grabbing

   a. Thumb and index finger

   b. Thumb and middle finger

Double-finger grabbing. Thumb and index finger.

Double-finger grabbing. Thumb and middle finger.

## B. Hand forms for cavity striking

1. Thumb

   a. Knuckle of thumb

   b. Tip of thumb

Knuckle of thumb.

Tip of thumb.

2. Fingertips
   a. Crane beak
   b. Eagle beak
   c. Fingertip hand
   d. Sword secret hand

Crane beak.

Eagle beak.

Fingertip hand.

Sword secret hand.

3. Palm
   a. Base of palm
   b. Edge of palm

Base of palm.

Edge of palm.

4. Fist
   a. Horizontal fist
   b. Vertical fist
   c. Back of fist
   d. Phoenix eye fist

Horizontal fist.

Vertical fist.

Back of fist.

Phoenix eye fist.

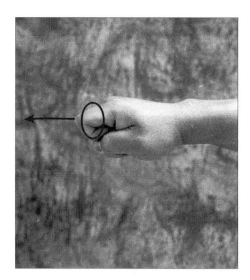

5. Wrist

   a.  Top side of wrist

Top side of wrist.

6. Elbow

   a.  External side of elbow

External side of elbow.

7. Foot
   a. Top of foot
   b. Heel
   c. Side of foot

Top of foot.

Heel.

Side of foot.

## 5-3. Qin Na and Cavity Press in Taiji Postures

The first posture, taiji beginning (*taiji qi shi,* 太極起勢), does not have actual combat applications. The purpose of this posture is to coordinate the mind, leading the qi to the lower dan tian. Therefore, often this posture is also called "sink qi to dan tian" (*qi chen dan tian,* 氣沈丹田). It is a preparatory movement that can bring the mind to your center and sink the qi firmly to the lower dan tian.

In addition, there are no combat applications for the last movement of taijiquan. This posture is commonly named "returning the taiji to its origin" (*taiji huan yuan,* 太極還原) or "lead the qi to return to its origin" (*yin qi gui yuan,* 引氣歸原). From the name, you can see that after practicing the entire taiji sequence, this posture is used to return the qi to its origin—the lower dan tian.

### 1. Grasp Sparrow's Tail (Lan Qiu Wei, 攬雀尾)

### A. Grasp Sparrow's Tail, Right (Lan Qiu Wei, You, 右)

### Movements

Turn your body to your right and move your right hand up with your left hand, slightly touching the middle portion of your right forearm.

**Analysis:**

This is an action of peng. The right arm is used as peng to neutralize the oncoming attack upward, and the left hand is used to support the right arm to enhance its neutralizing strength.

### Qin Na

### Technique #1. Use Wardoff Upward against Opponent's Elbow (Shang Peng Di Zhou, 上掤敵肘)

*Shang peng di zhou* is a technique that uses the movements of grasp sparrow's tail, right posture. In this technique, your left hand is used to pluck (cai, 採) your opponent's wrist while your right arm uses wardoff upward to lock his elbow.

Your left hand is used to pluck your opponent's wrist while your right arm uses wardoff upward to lock his elbow.

### Technique #2. Backward Upward Turning (Hou Shang Fan, 後上翻)

*Hou shang fan* is a technique that uses the movements of grasp sparrow's tail posture.

Situation: Your opponent attacks. First, use your right forearm wardoff against the opponent's attack, upward and to your right.

Immediately step your right leg to his right, and use your left hand to grab his right hand while circling your right elbow until it reaches his elbow.

Finally, twist his wrist with your left hand while lifting his elbow upward with your right elbow.

Alternative application: You may step your left leg behind him, and lock his right arm with your right hand and chest area while using your left arm to push the upper part of his head forward.

### Technique #3. Small Elbow Wrap (Xiao Chan Zhou, 小纏肘)

Xiao chan zhou is a technique that uses the movements of grasp sparrow's tail posture.

Situation: Your opponent attacks with his right hand. First, use your right forearm for an upward wardoff of your opponent's right hand attack.

Next, step your left leg to the front of his right leg, and hook and grab his right wrist with your right hand while placing your left forearm upward against his elbow.

Then bow forward, using the leverage of your left forearm and right hand to bend his arm, and then circle forward.

Finally, pull his body to your front while sweeping your left leg backward to make him fall.

**Technique #4. Arm Wraps around the Dragon's Neck (Bi Chan Long Jing, 臂纏龍頸)**

Bi chan long jing is a technique that uses the grasp sparrow's tail posture.

Situation: Your opponent uses a right hand attack. First, use your right forearm for an upward wardoff of your opponent's right hand attack.

Next, immediately hook your right hand down and grab his right wrist, and step your left leg behind his right leg while using your left forearm to push his neck backward.

Finally, lock his right arm with your chest and right hand while circling your left arm around his neck to lock him up.

From the above four examples, you can see that there are limited techniques that can be used directly from this posture. However, you will not be surprised to learn that this posture was originally designed to neutralize the opponent's attack or to set up and create an opportunity for the following technique.

**Cavity Press or Strike:**

When you use your right arm wardoff against the oncoming attack, you have exposed many of your opponent's cavities under his right arm.

This will offer you a great opportunity for the following attacks.

| Cavity name | Hand form(s) | Possible results |
|---|---|---|
| Jiquan (H-1, 極泉) | Sword secret | Cause heart attack |
| Qimen (Li-14, 期門) | Phoenix eye fist | Seal the breath and shock the liver |
| Riyue (GB-24, 日月) | Phoenix eye fist | Seal the breath and shock the liver |

Jiquan
(H-1)

Qimen (Li-14)
Riyue (GB-24)

Location of exposed cavity when using striking techniques in the arm wraps around the dragon's neck.

## B. Grasp Sparrow's Tail, Left (Zuo, 左)

### Movements

From the end of the grasp sparrow's tail, right posture, move both of your hands toward the center of your body and center yourself.

Then move your right hand downward and your left forearm upward and diagonally to your left using lie (rend) force.

## Analysis:

This action uses the pattern of lie force. This posture is commonly used right after grasp sparrow's tail, right. The power of lie on your left arm is generated from the balancing force of your right leg and right arm. One of the main forces is from the expanding of the chest, which is one of the two major bows in the body able to generate great power. The other bow is the torso.

## Qin Na

### Technique #1. Carry a Pole on the Shoulder (Jian Tiao Bian Dan, 肩挑扁擔)

Jian tiao bian dan is a technique that uses the movements of grasp sparrow's tail, left posture.

Situation: You use a right arm wardoff against your opponent's right hand attack. Immediately hook his arm down and grab his wrist while using your left arm to push his right post-arm.

Next, turn his right arm until his palm is facing upward while using your left shoulder to lift his post-arm upward from the tendons.

## Cavity Press or Strike:

Once you step your left leg behind his right leg, you have changed the distance, allowing you to use your elbow to strike the cavities. Generally, striking power generated from the elbow is much stronger than that of the fist.

When you attack, if possible, you should pull his right arm backward. This will enhance the striking power. Other than striking cavities, you may also use your left fist to strike upward to his nose or downward to his groin.

| Cavity name | Hand form(s) | Possible results |
| --- | --- | --- |
| Rugen (S-18, 乳根) | Elbow | Seal the breath |
| Qimen (Li-14, 期門) | Elbow | Seal the breath and shock the liver |
| Riyue (GB-24, 日月) | Elbow | Seal the breath and shock the liver |

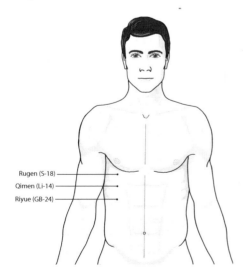

Rugen (S-18)
Qimen (Li-14)
Riyue (GB-24)

Locations of exposed cavities when using the striking techniques in carry a pole on the shoulder.

## 2. Wardoff (Peng, 掤)

### Movements

First, move your left arm upward with the fingers upward and the palm facing your face. Then rotate your left hand clockwise while turning your body to your left. While you are doing so, also draw your right leg back to your left leg while moving your right arm down and toward your body.

Next, step your right leg forward while pressing your left hand down and lifting your right forearm upward and forward.

### Analysis:

When peng is used for striking, the entire forearm is used to uproot the opponent or bounce him off his balance. Since the forearm cannot generate sharp, pointing pressure or penetrating power, it cannot be used for cavity striking. Normally, after you have used your left forearm to neutralize the oncoming attack, you use your right forearm to push his chest forward or upward. In fact, as explained in chapter 2, peng is also commonly used as a defensive action for neutralization.

Use your left forearm to neutralize the oncoming attack.

Use your right forearm to push his chest forward or upward.

## Qin Na

Please refer to chapter 3.

## Cavity Press or Strike:

None.

## 3. Rollback (Lu, 掤)

## Movements

The posture normally begins from one in which one of your arms is already extended forward.

Then sit backward and change your stance from bow and arrow stance into four six stance while moving both of your hands backward and to the side.

## Analysis:

Lu is commonly used to yield, lead, and neutralize the opponent's power. Although it is commonly considered a defensive action, you should understand that when the situation allows, lu can be used for offense.

### Qin Na

Please refer to chapter 3.

When you perform rollback, in order to immobilize your opponent's arm, your left hand and right hand can grab and press three cavities.

### Cavity Press or Strike:

| Cavity name | Hand form(s) | Possible results |
| --- | --- | --- |
| Shaohai (H-3, 少海) | Fingers | Cause numbness |
| Quchi (LI-11, 曲池) | Fingers | Cause numbness |
| Neiguan (P-6, 內關) | Fingers | Cause numbness or fainting |

Locations of exposed cavities when using the pressing techniques in rollback.

## 4. Press or Squeeze (Ji, 擠)

### Movements

In this taijiquan posture, when ji is executed, the left hand is on the wrist area of the right hand and is pressing.

### Analysis:

Ji can be used for both defense and offense. When ji is used for defense, it is commonly executed with both hands squeezing toward each other. However, when ji is used for attacking, it can be executed by either squeezing both hands toward each other or pressing forward. In the taijiquan sequence, it is commonly executed as forward pressing.

### Qin Na

Please refer to chapter 3.

### Cavity Press or Strike:

When you have a chance, use your left hand to press against your right wrist. You may then either press your opponent's chest or even use jerking jing to strike him.

| Cavity name | Hand form(s) | Possible results |
|---|---|---|
| Jiuwei (Co-15, 鳩尾) | Wrist | Seal the breath or heart attack |
| Zhongwan (Co-12, 中脘) | Wrist | Seal the breath and vomiting |

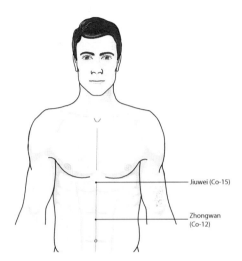

Location of exposed cavities when using pressing or striking techniques in ji.

## 5. Settle Down the Wrist (An, 按)

### Movements

### Analysis:

*An* can be used to seal the movement of your opponent's arm. It can also be used to neutralize the opponent's oncoming attack upward and then to strike his chest area, either with a single palm or double palms.

First, sit backward into a four six stance while raising both of your arms.

Then start to shift your weight to your front leg, and change into bow and arrow stance while pointing your fingers forward. Finally, just before both of your hands reach their maximum extension, settle your wrist and press forward.

Using *an* to seal the movement of your opponent's arm.

Using *an* to neutralize upward your opponent's attack.

Using *an* to strike the chest.

## Qin Na

Please refer to chapter 3.

## Cavity Press or Strike:

When *an* is used to attack, you can either use single or double hands to strike the cavity. In fact, the palm strike is one of the most common attacking techniques in taijiquan. There are many cavities that can be used for palm striking. We will introduce only some of the typical ones.

| Cavity name | Hand form(s) | Possible results |
|---|---|---|
| Ruzhong (S-17, 乳中) | Palm | Seal the breath |
| Rugen (S-18, 乳根) | Palm | Seal the breath |
| Jiuwei (Co-15, 鳩尾) | Palm | Seal the breath or heart attack |
| Zhongwan (Co-12, 中脘) | Palm | Seal the breath and vomiting |

Locations of exposed cavities when using striking techniques in *an*.

## 6. Single Whip (Dan Bian, 單鞭)

## Movements

The single whip (*dan bian*) posture includes three movements.

In the first movement, both of your hands are in front of your waist area and you use your body's turning momentum to move the hands to your left.

The second movement is moving your left hand down to face the right palm.

Then coil your right arm upward and backward.

In the third movement, turn your body to your left and deflect to the left, using your left arm.

## Analysis:

The first movement is the body's rotational movement. From the body's rotational momentum, the swinging power of the arms is generated. The second movement is from the coiling action of the right arm; the opponent's power is led upward and neutralized. Finally, the last movement is the action of *an*, which is applied to your opponent's chest.

Then step your left leg forward while pushing (*an*) your left hand forward.

## Qin Na

### Technique #1. Use Both Hands to Lead the Cow (Shuang Shou Qian Niu, 雙手牽牛)

*Shuang shou qian niu* is a technique that uses the single whip posture. In this qin na, the first movement of single whip, the rotation, is adopted.

Situation: You have a chance to use your left hand to grab your opponent's left wrist. Immediately use your right hand to lock and press his elbow. You can then lead him down to the ground or break his elbow.

## Technique #2. Diagonal Flying (Xie Fei Shi, 斜飛式)

*Xie fei shi* is a technique that uses the movements of the single whip posture. This qin na uses the second movement of single whip, coiling, to execute the technique.

Situation: Your opponent uses his right hand to punch you. Coil your right hand around his right wrist.

Next, grab his right wrist with your right hand, step your left leg behind his right leg, and use your left arm to push against his neck while locking his right arm in front of your chest.

## Technique #3. Roast Peking Duck (Bei Ping Kao Ya, 北平烤鴨)

*Bei Ping kao ya* is a technique that uses the single whip posture.

Situation: Your opponent punches you with his right fist. Immediately intercept with your left forearm and circle around his wrist and grab it.

While you are doing so, also move your left hand upward to keep his right arm bent. Then rotate his right palm until his palm faces upward and use your left and right hands to lock his arm upward.

### Cavity Press or Strike:

In the first movement, you are grabbing and leading his arm. In this grabbing, three cavities are usually used. In the final movement, it is an action of *an*.

The common places for executing this *an* are on the chest area.

| Cavity name | Hand form(s) | Possible results |
| --- | --- | --- |
| Shaohai (H-3, 少海) | Fingers | Cause numbness |
| Quchi (LI-11, 曲池) | Fingers | Cause numbness |
| Neiguan (P-6, 內關) | Fingers | Cause numbness or fainting |
| Ruzhong (S-17, 乳中) | Palm | Seal the breath |
| Rugen (S-18, 乳根) | Palm | Seal the breath |

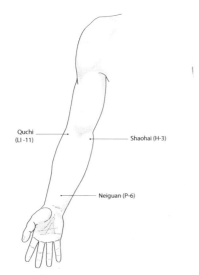

Locations of exposed cavities when executing grabbing movements in single whip.

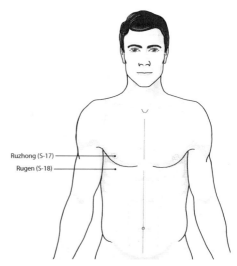

Locations of exposed cavities when executing *an*, using single whip.

## 7. Lift Hands and Lean Forward (Ti Shou Shang Shi, 提手上勢)

### Movements

First, move both of your hands toward your center.

Then extend your right arm up and out while stepping your right leg forward, and touch the ground with your heel.

## Analysis:

In this posture, the right arm's upward and forward lifting are used to intercept the attack, and the right leg is used to kick the opponent's knee or groin. In addition, the left hand on the front of the chest is ready for an attack.

## Qin Na

### Technique #1. Heaven King Supports the Pagoda (Tian Wang Tuo Ta, 天王托塔)

*Tian wang tuo ta* is a technique that uses the lift hands and lean forward posture.

Situation: Your opponent punches you with his left fist. Immediately raise your right arm to intercept his attack.

Next, coil your left arm up to his elbow while using your left hand to grab his left wrist.

Finally, step your right leg beside his left leg, and use the leverage generated from both of your hands to lock him up.

## Cavity Press or Strike:

The right arm's upward and forward movement is an interception. The right leg's movement is designed to either kick the knee or groin.

The left hand hidden underneath the right elbow is for a follow-up attack.

| Cavity name | Hand form(s) | Possible results |
|---|---|---|
| Ruzhong (S-17, 乳中) | Palm or fist | Seal the breath |
| Rugen (S-18, 乳根) | Palm or fist | Seal the breath |
| Jiuwei (Co-15, 鳩尾) | Palm or fist | Seal the breath or heart attack |
| Zhongwan (Co-12, 中脘) | Palm or fist | Seal the breath and vomiting |

Locations of exposed cavities when using striking techniques in lift hands and raise forward.

## 8. The Crane Spreads Its Wings (Bai He Liang Chi, 白鶴亮翅)

**Movements**

First, move both of your hands toward your center.

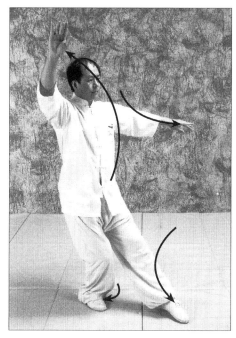

Then open them outward while touching the ground with your left toes.

### Analysis:

This posture includes two movements: one is closing and the other is opening. The movement is generated from the chest instead of just the arms. Therefore, the upward spreading has a feeling of wardoff (peng, 掤). The stance on your left leg is called false stance because it can be used for easy and sudden kicks.

## Qin Na

### Technique #1. Left Right Cross Elbow (Zuo You Jiao Zhou, 左右交肘)

Zuo you jiao zhou is a technique that uses the movements of the grasp sparrow's tail posture.

Situation: Your opponent punches you with his right fist. First, intercept the punch with your right hand.

Then pluck it downward.

In this situation, it is very easy for your opponent to attack you with his left hand.

When this happens, immediately use your left forearm to intercept his left hand punch and pluck it downward. Then rotate both of his arms to lock him up.

## Technique #2. The Crane Spreads Its Wings (Bai He Liang Chi, 白鶴亮翅)

Bai he liang chi is a technique that uses the grasp sparrow's tail posture.

Situation: Your opponent punches you with his right fist. First, use your left hand to cover his punch.

Next, grab his right wrist with your left hand and immediately use both hands to twist his wrist counterclockwise.

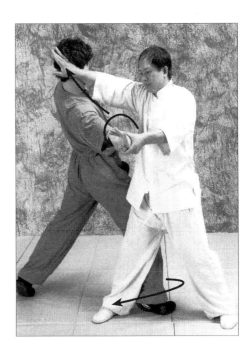

Finally, continue your left hand's twisting while using your right forearm to push his neck to your right. This will offer you good leverage for locking.

## Cavity Press or Strike:

The arms' closing and opening is used to seal or to lock. There is no striking purpose.

There is no striking purpose from the arms closing and opening, but you may have set up an opportunity for kicking.

Your left leg can be used to kick the lower part of your opponent's body.

| Cavity name | Hand form(s) | Possible results |
|---|---|---|
| Qihai (Co-6, 氣海) | Heel | Death |
| Groin (Organ, 下陰) | Toes or heel | Death |

Qihai (Co-6)

Groin

Locations of exposed cavities when using kicking techniques in crane spreads its wings.

## 9. Brush Knee and Step Forward (Lou Xi Yao Bu, 摟膝拗步)

### Movements

First, turn your body to your right while rotating your right hand clockwise and also pushing your left forearm to your right.

Next, step your left leg forward and coil your left hand downward.

### Analysis:

This posture includes two major parts. The first part is the neutralization and then coiling down the left arm, and the second part is the right hand's *an*.

Finally, use your right hand to press forward (*an*).

## Qin Na

### Technique #1. Reverse Elbow Wrap (Fan Chan Zhou, 反纏肘)

Fan chan zhou is a technique that uses the movements of the brush knee and step forward posture.

(This technique uses the first part of the brush knee and step forward posture's movements.) Situation: Your opponent punches you with his right fist. First, intercept with your right forearm while using your left forearm to seal his right elbow.

Next, step your left leg behind his right leg while coiling your left hand around his right arm until it reaches his post-arm near the elbow.

Finally, use the leverage generated from your left elbow and hand to press and circle him down to the ground.

## Technique #2. Small Elbow Wrap (Xiao Chan Zhou, 小纏肘)

Xiao chan zhou is a technique that uses the movements of the brush knee and step forward posture.

Situation: Your opponent punches you with his right fist. Use your right forearm to intercept the attack while using your left forearm to seal his elbow.

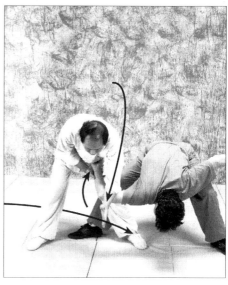

Next, step your left leg to the front of his right leg, grabbing his right wrist with your right hand and pressing his elbow down with your left hand.

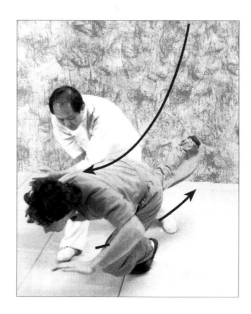

Finally, sweep your left leg backward while using the leverage generated from your right hand and left forearm to swing him down to the ground.

## Technique #3. Both Hands Twist the Neck (Shuang Shou Niu Jing, 雙手扭頸)

*Shuang shou niu jing* is a technique that uses the movements of the brush knee and step forward posture.

Situation: Your opponent punches you with his right fist. Immediately neutralize his attack.

Step your left leg behind his right leg while moving your right hand to his chin and your left hand behind his head.

Then use the leverage generated from both of your hands to break his neck.

## Cavity Press or Strike:

Neutralize the attack.

Step your left leg behind his right leg to keep away from his left hand while using your left hand to push the center of his back forward and using your right palm to strike his chest area. To obtain a better angle for the attack, you should focus on the front upper-body area.

| Cavity name | Hand form(s) | Possible results |
|---|---|---|
| Tiantu (Co-22, 天突) | Thumb | Seal the breath |
| Yingchuang (S-16, 膺窗) | Palm or phoenix eye fist | Seal the breath |
| Ruzhong (S-17, 乳中) | Palm or phoenix eye fist | Seal the breath |
| Rugen (S-18, 乳根) | Palm or phoenix eye fist | Seal the breath |
| Jiuwei (Co-15, 鳩尾) | Palm | Seal the breath or heart attack |
| Zhongwan (Co-12, 中脘) | Palm | Seal the breath and vomiting |

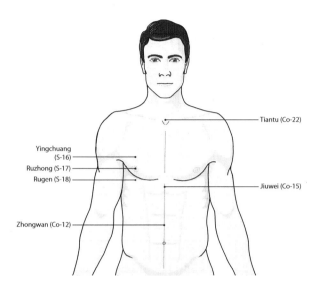

Tiantu (Co-22)

Yingchuang (S-16)

Ruzhong (S-17)

Rugen (S-18)

Jiuwei (Co-15)

Zhongwan (Co-12)

Locations of exposed cavities when using striking techniques in brush knee and step forward.

## 10. Play the Guitar (Shou Hui Pi Pa, 手揮琵琶)

### Movements

First, move your right leg next to your left leg while lifting your right arm upward.

Next, step your left leg forward and enter a false stance while moving your left hand under your right elbow. Continue extending your left hand forward and moving your right hand to your left armpit area.

## Analysis:

Your right arm's upward movement is used to neutralize the oncoming attack upward. Your left hand's following movement is to repel your opponent's arm to the side, and your left leg's stepping is used for kicking. After your neutralization and repelling, your right hand is ready for further attack.

## Qin Na

### Technique #1. Heaven King Supports the Pagoda (Tian Wang Tuo Ta, 天王托塔)

Tian wang tuo ta is a technique that uses the movements of the play the guitar posture.

Situation: Your opponent attacks you with his right hand. Immediately use your right forearm to intercept his right forearm while placing your left forearm under his right elbow.

Next, grab his right wrist with your right hand and use the leverage generated from your right hand and left forearm to lock his right elbow.

Alternative application: Intercept his right arm.

Use your left hand to push his elbow upward to lock it.

### Technique #2: Forward Upward Turning (Qian Shang Fan, 前上翻)

Qian shang fan is a technique that uses the play the guitar posture.

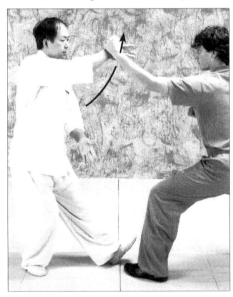

Situation: Your opponent punches you with his left hand. Immediately step your right leg backward and lift your right arm upward to intercept his attack.

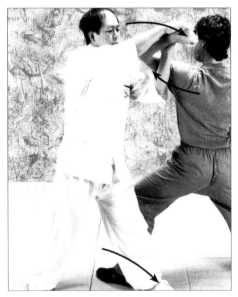

Next, step your left leg behind his left leg, and use your left forearm to pull his left elbow toward you while pushing his wrist toward him with your right hand.

Finally, lock his left arm with your left arm while pushing the upper back of his head forward to lock his arm firmly.

## Cavity Press or Strike:

Neutralize the attack with your right arm.

Grab his right wrist with your right hand while locking his elbow with your left hand. From this setup, you may then kick the lower part of his body.

Alternative strike: Step your left leg behind his right leg to avoid his left hand's attack while using your left hand to seal his elbow and using your right fist to attack him.

| Cavity name | Hand form(s) | Possible results |
| --- | --- | --- |
| Qihai (Co-6, 氣海) | Heel | Death |
| Groin (Organ, 下陰) | Toes or heel | Death |
| Jiquan (H-1, 極泉) | Sword secret | Cause a heart attack |
| Ruzhong (S-17, 乳中) | Palm or phoenix eye fist | Seal the breath |
| Rugen (S-18, 乳根) | Palm or phoenix eye fist | Seal the breath |
| Qimen (Li-14, 期門) | Phoenix eye fist | Seal the breath and shock the liver |
| Riyue (GB-24, 日月) | Phoenix eye fist | Seal the breath and shock the liver |

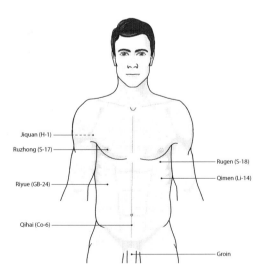

Locations of exposed cavities when using striking or kicking techniques in play the guitar.

## 11. Twist Body and Circle Fist (Pie Shen Chui, 撇身捶)

### Movements

First, turn your body to your left while lowering your right arm and moving it toward your left.

Next, turn your body to your right, circling your right arm upward and then downward.

### Analysis:

Your right arm's downward movement is used to neutralize the lower attack to your left, and the right arm's upward and forward circling is used to strike the opponent.

Finally, move your right hand to the right side of your waist while covering downward with your left forearm.

## Qin Na

### Technique #1: Large Elbow Wrap (Da Chan Zhou, 大纏肘)

*Da chan zhou* is a technique that uses the movements of the twist body and circle fist posture.

Situation: Your opponent attacks your lower body with his right hand. Immediately use your right forearm to neutralize his attack to your left while also using your left hand to grab his right wrist.

Next, reposition yourself while circling your right arm upward to bend his right arm.

Finally, place your right hand on his post-arm near the elbow and use the leverage generated from both of your hands to lock him down to the ground.

**Cavity Press or Strike:**

After your right arm's neutralization, you can easily circle your right hand upward and then forward to strike him.

| Cavity name | Hand form(s) | Possible results |
| --- | --- | --- |
| Shangen (M-HN-4, 山根) | Back of fist | Fainting, nose bleed |
| Renzhong (Gv-26, 人中) | Back of fist | Fainting |

Shangen (M-HN-4)

Renzhong (Gv-26)

Locations of exposed cavities when using striking techniques in twist body and circle fist.

## 12. Step Forward, Deflect Downward, Parry, and Punch (Shang Bu Ban Lan Chui, 上步扳攔捶)

### Movements

First, turn your body to your right while covering downward with your left arm.

Then step your left leg forward while punching your right hand forward.

## Analysis:

Your left arm's covering is used to neutralize the attack downward. Right after the neutralization, immediately punch your right fist forward for an attack.

### Qin Na

### Technique #1: Step Forward and Deflect Downward (Shang Bu Ban Zhou, 上步扳肘)

*Shang bu ban zhou* is a technique that uses the movements of the step forward and deflect downward posture.

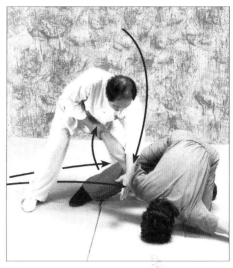

Situation: Your opponent attacks you with his right fist. Immediately intercept it with your right forearm and then grab his wrist while covering with your left forearm on his elbow.

Next, step your left leg behind his right leg, bow forward and use the leverage of both of your hands to lock his arm, and lead him down to the ground.

## Cavity Press or Strike:

Right after you cover his attack, you may continue to lead his right arm to your left while stepping your left leg behind his right leg to avoid his left hand's attack and using your right fist to attack his abdominal area.

Alternative strike: You may strike the groin.

| Cavity name | Hand form(s) | Possible results |
|---|---|---|
| Qimen (Li-14, 期門) | Fist | Seal the breath and shock the liver |
| Riyue (GB-24, 日月) | Fist | Seal the breath and shock the liver |
| Groin (Organ, 下陰) | Palm | Death |

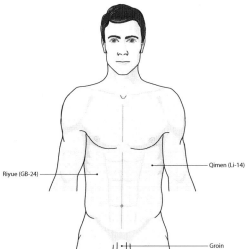

Locations of exposed cavities when using striking techniques in step forward, deflect downward, parry, and punch.

## 13. Seal Tightly (Ru Feng Si Bi, 如封似閉)

### Movements

First, slide your left hand inward along your right arm until you reach the right elbow.

Next, coil to the bottom of the elbow and then outward.

Keep extending your left hand forward while withdrawing your right hand and sitting back into four six stance.

Finally, strike your right palm forward and change the stance into bow and arrow stance.

### Analysis:

This posture is designed for use against grabbing. While you try to free your right arm, you are also coiling your left hand around your right arm until you reach your opponent's body, either to grab him or to lock him. This will provide you with an opportunity to attack.

## Qin Na

### Technique #1: Roast Peking Duck (Bei Ping Kao Ya, 北平烤鴨)

Bei Ping kao ya is a technique that uses movements of the seal tightly posture.

Situation: Your opponent uses his right hand to grab your right wrist.

Immediately circle your right hand counterclockwise to reverse the grabbing while extending your left hand under his right arm.

Next, step your left leg behind his right leg, grab his right wrist, and continue extending your left arm until it reaches his neck.

Finally, rotate his arm until his palm is facing up and press it downward while straightening out your left arm to lock him up.

### Technique #2: Low Outward Wrist Press (Xia Wai Ya Wan, 下外壓腕)

*Xia wai ya wan* is a technique that uses the movements of the seal tightly posture.

Situation: You have an opportunity to grab your opponent's right wrist with your right hand. Immediately move your left arm under his right arm.

Next, step your left leg behind his right leg while coiling your left hand until it reaches his elbow.

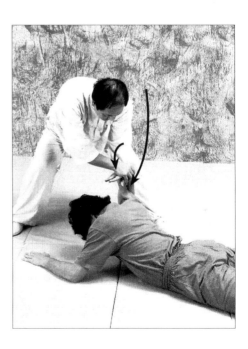

Finally, bend his wrist while continuing to lock his right elbow until his body is on the ground.

## Cavity Press or Strike:

Your left hand's coiling is trying to reach your opponent to catch his arm while you try to free your right hand.

If you are able to lock his right arm, you may use your left hand to press the cavities beside his neck to seal his breath.

Alternative strike: Right after you have grabbed his right arm with your left hand, you may immediately use your right hand to attack his chest area.

| Cavity name | Hand form(s) | Possible results |
|---|---|---|
| Tianrong (SI-17, 天容) | Thumb | Seal the artery |
| Jianjing (GB-21, 肩井) | Grabbing | Fainting or numbness |
| Ruzhong (S-17, 乳中) | Palm | Seal the breath |
| Rugen (S-18, 乳根) | Palm | Seal the breath |
| Qimen (Li-14, 期門) | Fist | Seal the breath and shock the liver |
| Riyue (GB-24, 日月) | Fist | Seal the breath and shock the liver |

Location of exposed cavity when using pressing techniques in seal tightly.

Location of exposed cavity when using grabbing techniques in seal tightly.

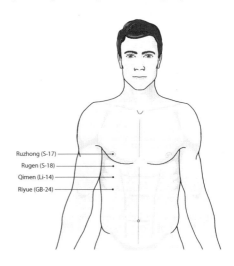

Locations of exposed cavities when using striking techniques in seal tightly.

## 14. Embrace Tiger and Return to the Mountain (Bao Hu Gui Shan, 抱虎歸山)

### Movements

Cross both of your arms in front of you until they are as high as your head.

Next, squat on your right leg and continue to circle both of your arms down.

### Analysis:

This is an opening and closing action in taijiquan. These kinds of actions are commonly used to seal or to immobilize the arm movement of your opponent.

Finally, move both of your arms in front of your chest and stand upward in horse stance.

## Qin Na

### Technique #1: Embrace Tiger and Return to the Mountain (Bao Hu Gui Shan, 抱虎歸山)

Bao hu gui shan is a technique that uses the movements of the embrace tiger and return to the mountain posture.

Situation: Your opponent tries to use both of his hands to grab you. Immediately move your arms upward to intercept his two arms.

Next, step both of your legs toward him to get closer while circling both of his arms to his back.

Finally, use your chin to press his right upper chest while holding both of his arms behind him.

## Technique #2: Large Python Coils the Neck (Da Mang Chan Jing, 大蟒纏頸)

*Da mang chan jing* is a technique that uses the movements of the embrace tiger and return to the mountain posture.

Situation: Your opponent punches you with his right arm. Immediately use your right hand to seal the punch upward.

Next, step your left leg behind him while inserting your left hand under his armpit, and try to reach his neck.

Finally, use your left hand to lock his neck while lifting his right arm.

### Technique #3: Large Ape Bends the Branch (Da Yuan Pan Zhi, 大猿攀枝)

*Da yuan pan zhi* is a technique that uses the movements of the embrace tiger and return to the mountain posture.

Situation: Your opponent uses his right fist to punch you. Immediately intercept it with your right forearm and then pluck his hand downward.

In this case, it is very possible that your opponent will execute a second punch from his left hand. Once you notice this, immediately use your left forearm to intercept it upward and grab it.

Next, step your left leg behind him and circle both of his arms behind him.

Finally, use your right leg to push his sacrum forward to lock him in place.

## Cavity Press or Strike:

The major effectiveness of this posture comes from the section that provides the seal. The seal provides the opportunity for grabbing or striking.

After the seal, immediately step your left leg beside his right leg while using both of your hands to attack your opponent's groin area.

| Cavity name | Hand form(s) | Possible results |
|---|---|---|
| Groin (Organ, 下陰) | Grabbing | Death |

## 15. Fist Under the Elbow (Zhou Di Kan Chui, 肘底看捶)

### Movements

Begin from the end of the single whip posture.

Move your right leg next to the left leg while moving your right hand above your head.

Next, step your right leg to your right.

Then shift your weight to your right leg, and at the same time cover downward with your right arm.

## Analysis:

This posture is a training for stepping into the opponent's left empty door. When stepping your right leg to your right and then turning to the left, you have occupied the space on your opponent's left side, which allows you to attack. Your right hand's movement is to coordinate the stepping in protecting yourself, and your left hand's extending movement is for attacking. If you pay attention to the name of this posture, you can see that the meaning is "beware of the fist under the elbow." That means the right fist under the left elbow is used to attack.

Finally, extend your left arm above your right hand while stepping your left leg forward into a false stance.

## Qin Na

### Technique #1: Left Right Cross Elbow (Zuo You Jiao Zhou, 左右交肘)

Zuo you jiao zhou is a technique that uses the movements of the fist under the elbow posture.

Situation: Your opponent attacks you with his right hand. First, step your right leg to your right to dodge the attack while covering his forearm with your right arm.

Next, grab his right wrist with your right hand and pull it down. This will offer your opponent an opportunity to execute his second punch with his left hand. In this case, raise your left arm up to block his punch while moving your left leg forward.

Finally, rotate both of his arms and use his right arm to lock his left arm in place. His left arm should be kept straight.

**Technique #2: Twist the Wrist Under the Elbow (Zhou Di Zhi Wan, 肘底制腕)**

*Zhou di zhi wan* is a technique that uses the movements of the fist under the elbow posture.

Situation: You discover your opponent is extending his left hand to grab you. Immediately cover his left fingers with your right hand and twist them counterclockwise.

Then step your left leg behind his left leg, continue to twist his left fingers, and push them toward his armpit while using your left elbow to press his neck. This will cause great pain in his pinkie's tendon.

## Technique #3: Daoist Greets with Hands (Dao Zi Zuo Ji, 道子作揖)

*Dao zi zuo ji* is a technique that uses the movements of the fist under the elbow posture. This qin na uses the right hand's cover and left arm's lifting motion from the posture.

Situation: Your opponent attacks you with his right hand. Use your right forearm to intercept his right forearm while using your left forearm to intercept his right elbow.

Then step your left leg behind his right leg, and press his forearm downward while using your left elbow to lift up his elbow to lock him.

## Cavity Press or Strike:

There are three attacking opportunities made available from this posture. The first one is the left leg's kicking.

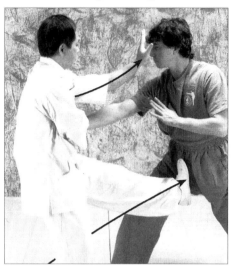

The first opportunity is the left leg's kick. The second is usually the left hand's attack to his face.

Often, this face strike is a fake attack that is used to distract your opponent or to tempt him to block upward. This will create an opportunity for the third attack, which is the hidden fist under the left elbow.

| Cavity name | Hand form(s) | Possible results |
|---|---|---|
| Qihai (Co-6, 氣海) | Heel | Death |
| Groin (Organ, 下陰) | Toes or heel | Death |
| Tiantu (Co-22, 天突) | Sword secret | Seal the breath |
| Jiuwei (Co-15, 鳩尾) | Palm or fist | Seal the breath or heart attack |
| Zhongwan (Co-12, 中脘) | Palm or fist | Seal the breath and vomiting |
| Ruzhong (S-17, 乳中) | Palm or phoenix eye fist | Seal the breath |
| Rugen (S-18, 乳根) | Palm or phoenix eye fist | Seal the breath |
| Qimen (Li-14, 期門) | Phoenix eye fist or fist | Seal the breath and shock the liver |
| Riyue (GB-24, 日月) | Phoenix eye fist or fist | Seal the breath and shock the liver |

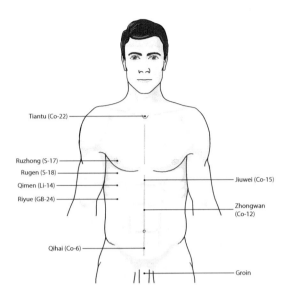

Tiantu (Co-22)

Ruzhong (S-17)
Rugen (S-18)
Qimen (Li-14)
Riyue (GB-24)

Jiuwei (Co-15)

Zhongwan (Co-12)

Qihai (Co-6)

Groin

Locations of exposed cavities when using kicking or striking techniques in fist under the elbow.

## 16. Step Back and Repulse Monkey (Dao Nian Hou, 倒撺猴)

### Movements

In the beginning posture your left hand extends forward, your right hand is on your right waist, and you are standing in a four six stance.

Next, stand on your right leg, and rotate your left hand until the palm is facing upward while circling your right hand to the right ear area.

Then turn your right foot until the toes are facing forward.

Finally, step your left leg backward, pushing your right hand forward while pulling your left hand backward.

## Analysis:

Your left hand's turning is against a grabbing. From this rotational action, you will be able to free your hand. Your stepping backward is used as a yield or withdrawal. Often, this stepping can also be used as a strategic movement. Naturally, your right hand's forward pushing (*an*, 按) is used for striking.

## Qin Na

### Technique #1: Twist the Wrist and Push the Neck (Niu Wan Tui Jing, 扭腕推頸)

*Niu wan tui jing* is a technique that uses the movements of the step back and repulse monkey posture.

Situation: Your opponent punches you with his right fist. Immediately step your right leg backward while using your left forearm to cover the punch.

Next, use both hands to twist his right wrist.

Finally, continue his wrist's twisting with your left hand, step your right leg behind his right leg while pushing your right hand against his neck. This will lock his arm in position.

## Cavity Press or Strike:

Your left hand's twisting can either be used to escape from your opponent's grabbing or to control his wrist. Once you have controlled your opponent's wrist, then you will be able to use the other hand to attack the front of his body.

| Cavity name | Hand form(s) | Possible results |
|---|---|---|
| Tiantu (Co-22, 天突) | Sword secret | Seal the breath |
| Jiuwei (Co-15, 鳩尾) | Palm or fist | Seal the breath or heart attack |
| Zhongwan (Co-12, 中脘) | Palm or fist | Seal the breath and vomiting |
| Ruzhong (S-17, 乳中) | Palm or phoenix eye fist | Seal the breath |
| Rugen (S-18, 乳根) | Palm or phoenix eye fist | Seal the breath |
| Qimen (Li-14, 期門) | Phoenix eye fist or fist | Seal the breath and shock the liver |
| Riyue (GB-24, 日月) | Phoenix eye fist or fist | Seal the breath and shock the liver |

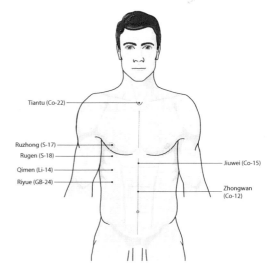

Locations of exposed cavities when using striking techniques in step back and repulse monkey.

## 17. Diagonal Flying (Xie Fei Shi, 斜飛勢)

### Movements

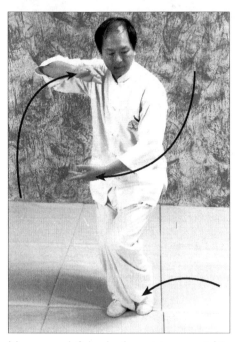

Move your left leg back next to your right leg while circling your left hand down and your right hand up.

Then step your left leg forward while splitting your arms diagonally.

## Analysis:

This is a combination of wardoff (peng) and rend (lie). The downward and upward diagonal movements are able to generate good leverage for the rend power.

### Qin Na

### Technique #1: Diagonal Flying to Support the Arm (Xie Fei Cheng Bi, 斜飛撐臂)

*Xie fei cheng bi* is a technique that uses the movements of the diagonal flying posture.

Situation: Your opponent punches you with his right hand. Use your right hand to intercept, and then coil to the right.

## Cavity Press or Strike:

Next, step your left leg behind his right leg, grab his right wrist, and pull it down while using your left shoulder to lock his right post-arm.

Your right hand's grabbing and pulling his right arm downward are to expose his head area to your attack.

For example, when the throat is chopped, the breath can be sealed, and when the side of the neck is chopped, the artery can be sealed.

| Cavity name | Hand form(s) | Possible results |
|---|---|---|
| Throat | Edge of palm | Seal the breath |
| Futu (LI-18, 伏兔) | Edge of palm | Seal the artery |
| Taiyang (M-HN-9, 太陽) | Phoenix eye fist | Death (rupture the artery) |
| Jiache (S-6, 頰車) | Back of fist | Fainting |

Locations of exposed cavities when using striking techniques in diagonal flying.

### 18. Pick Up Needle from Sea Bottom (Hai Di Lao Zhen, 海底撈針)

**Movements**

Begin from the movement in which your right arm is pushing forward and your left hand is beside your left waist.

Move your left leg backward and enter a false stance while lifting your right arm upward and your left hand in front of your chest.

### Analysis:

When your opponent is attacking your chest, use your right arm to intercept the attack upward to expose his lower body for your strike. Your left hand pushes his elbow to immobilize his arm's movement, which offers you an opportunity for your right hand attack. Often, after the right arm's upward intercepting, it is used to pluck (cai, 採) the opponent's wrist and pull it down to expose his head or to make him lose balance.

Finally, sink your right arm downward and at the same time squat into a low posture.

## Qin Na

### Technique #1. Upward Pushing Enemy's Elbow (Shang Tui Di Zhou, 上推敵肘)

*Shang tui di zhou* is a technique that uses the movements of the pick up needle from sea bottom posture.

Situation: Your opponent attacks you with his right hand. Immediately withdraw your left leg while using your right arm to intercept the attack upward and your left hand to seal his elbow.

Then step your left leg forward and pull his right wrist down while pushing his elbow upward with your left hand. In this case, you have locked his right arm. If you use power, you can break his elbow.

### Technique #2. Step Forward and Deflect Downward (Shang Bu Ban Zhou, 上步扳肘)

Shang bu ban zhou is a technique that uses the movements of the pick up needle from sea bottom posture.

Situation: Your opponent attacks you with his right fist. Immediately intercept it with your right forearm and then grab his wrist while pushing your left hand upward on his elbow.

Next, reposition yourself, bow forward, and use the leverage of both of your hands to lock his arm down to the ground.

### Cavity Press or Strike:

Right after you have intercepted your opponent's attack upward, you will have opened up many cavities on the forward right side of his body for your attack.

This will naturally include the left leg's kicking to his knee.

You may use your left hand to seal his right arm while using your right hand to attack the side of his body.

| Cavity name | Hand form(s) | Possible results |
|---|---|---|
| Qimen (Li-14, 期門) | Fist | Seal the breath and shock the liver |
| Riyue (GB-24, 日月) | Fist | Seal the breath and shock the liver |
| Groin (Organ) | Palm | Death |

Locations of exposed cavities when using striking techniques in pick up needle from sea bottom.

### 19. Fan Back (Shan Tong Bei, 扇通背)

**Movements**

First, move your left leg back and stand in false stance while placing your left hand in front of you and your right hand above and in front of your head.

Next, step your left leg forward and push both of your hands forward with your body.

## Analysis:

The first movement is used for yielding and the second movement can be used either for sealing or for pushing.

## Qin Na

### Technique #1. Forward Upward Turning (Qian Shang Fan, 前上翻)

Qian shang fan is a technique that uses the movements of the fan back posture.

Situation: Your opponent punches you with his right hand. Immediately step your left leg backward and lift your right arm to intercept his attack while using your left hand to seal his elbow.

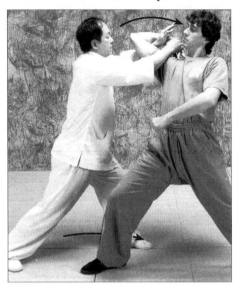

Next, step your left leg behind his right leg, and use your left forearm to pull his right elbow toward you while pushing his wrist toward him with your right hand.

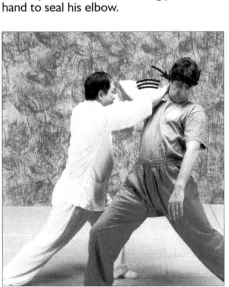

Finally, lock his right arm with your left arm while pushing the upper back of his head forward to lock his arm firmly.

## Technique #2. Daoist Greets with Hands (Dao Zi Zuo Ji, 道子作揖)

Dao zi zuo ji is a technique that uses the movements of the fan back posture.

Situation: Your opponent punches you with his right hand. Withdraw your left leg while using your right forearm to intercept his attack upward and your left hand to seal his elbow.

Then use the leverage of your left and right hands to lock his right arm.

### Cavity Press or Strike:

When your opponent's arm is blocked upward, his armpit and the right side of his body will be exposed for your attack.

Naturally, you may also use your left hand to grab the tendons under his armpit to numb his arm and impede its movement.

| Cavity name | Hand form(s) | Possible results |
|---|---|---|
| Jiquan (H-1, 極泉) | Sword secret | Cause a heart attack |
| Yuanye (GB-22, 淵腋) | Phoenix eye fist | Seal the breath |
| Dabao (Sp-21, 大包) | Phoenix eye fist | Seal the breath |

Yuanye (GB-22)

Dabao (Sp-21)

Locations of exposed cavities when using striking techniques in fan back.

### 20. Wave Hands in Clouds (Yun Shou, 雲手)

## Movements

First, turn your body to your right while pressing your left hand downward.

Next, raise your right forearm.

## Analysis:

Both of your hands' actions are used to seal or to lock your opponent's arm. Your body's turning is to throw your opponent off balance or to break his elbow.

Then turn your body to your right.

## Qin Na

### Technique #1. Cloud Hands to Lock the Elbow (Yun Shou Jia Zhou, 雲手架肘)

*Yun shou jia zhou* is a technique that uses the movements of the wave hands in clouds posture.

Situation: Your opponent attacks you with his right hand. Immediately use your left forearm to intercept.

Next, step your left leg to his right side while pressing his wrist down with your left hand and propping up his right post-arm or elbow with your right forearm.

Finally, push his wrist forward, and pull his post-arm or elbow inward while pressing your right elbow to the side of his chest to lock him up.

## Technique #2. Large Elbow Wrap (Da Chan Zhou, 大纏肘)

Da chan zhou is a technique that uses the movements of the wave hands in clouds posture.

Situation: Your opponent attacks you with his right hand. Use your left forearm to intercept his punch and then press his arm downward while using your right hand to lock his elbow.

Next, step your left leg behind his right leg and raise your right arm to bend his right arm.

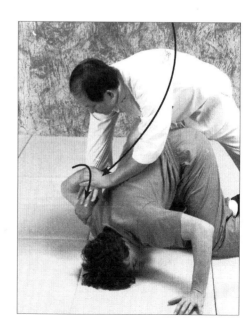

Finally, step your right leg backward while using the leverage generated from both of your hands to lock him down to the ground.

## Cavity Press or Strike:

Once you have locked your opponent's arm with both of your hands, you may also use your right elbow to strike the sides of his upper body.

In addition, the lower section of his body will also be exposed for your knee attack.

| Cavity name | Hand form(s) | Possible results |
|---|---|---|
| Qihai (Co-6, 氣海) | Knee | Death |
| Groin (Organ, 下陰) | Knee | Death |
| Yuanye (GB-22, 淵腋) | Elbow | Seal the breath |
| Dabao (Sp-21, 大包) | Elbow | Seal the breath |

Yuanye
(GB-22)

Dabao
(Sp-21)

Qihai
(Co-6)

Locations of exposed cavities when using striking or kicking techniques in wave hands in clouds.

### 21. Stand High to Search Out the Horse (Gao Tan Ma, 高探馬)

**Movements**

Begin with your right hand pressing forward.

Withdraw your left leg and stand in false stance while moving your right hand to the front and slightly above your head and your left hand in front of your chest.

## Analysis:

This movement is just like the first movement of the fan back posture, which is used to neutralize the upper-body attack. The left leg is set up for a kicking technique.

Situation: Your opponent attacks your upper body with his right hand. First, neutralize his attack.

This sets up your left leg for kicking.

## Qin Na

Please refer to posture nineteen, fan back.

## Cavity Press or Strike:

Please refer to posture nineteen, fan back.

### 22. Toe Kick (Ti Tui, 踢腿)

## Movements

First, turn your body to your left while crossing your arms in front of your chest.

Next, open both of your arms and kick your right toes out to your right.

## Analysis:

The arms' closing and opening are used to intercept the opponent's attack upward, which will expose the opponent's middle and lower body to your kicking.

## Qin Na

No qin na applications.

## Cavity Press or Strike:

Although the name is called toe kick in taijiquan, if you use the toes to kick, the only place you can attack is the groin. However, if you also use the side of your foot or your heel to kick, then you may kick the side of the ribs to rupture the liver.

| Cavity name | Hand form(s) | Possible results |
|---|---|---|
| Qimen (Li-14, 期門) | Side of foot or heel | Seal the breath and rupture the liver |
| Riyue (GB-24, 日月) | Side of foot or heel | Seal the breath and rupture the liver |
| Groin (Organ, 下陰) | Toes | Death |

Locations of exposed cavities when using kicking techniques in toe kick.

## 23. Heel Kick (Deng Tui, 蹬腿)

### Movements

First, cross both of your arms in front of your chest.

Next, open both of your arms and kick your heel out in front of you.

### Analysis:

Both of your hands are used to grab your opponent's arm or even clothes, and then the heel is used to kick the center of his body. Naturally, if the distance is too short, you may also use your knee to strike.

### Qin Na

### Technique #1. Fair Lady Picks the Peach (Xian Niu Zhai Tao, 仙女摘桃)

*Xian niu zhai tao* is a technique that uses the movements of the heel kick posture.

Situation: Your opponent intends to use both of his hands to grab you or both palms to strike your chest. Immediately step your right leg backward while using both of your hands to grab his fingers on both hands.

Next, turn his left fingers clockwise and his right fingers counterclockwise, and bend them down.

Under this locking situation, you may be able to use your right leg to kick him.

## Cavity Press or Strike:

Once you have used both of your arms to intercept both of your opponent's hands, his lower body will be exposed for your kicking.

| Cavity name | Hand form(s) | Possible results |
| --- | --- | --- |
| Zhongwan (Co-12, 中脘) | Heel | Seal the breath and vomiting |
| Qihai (Co-6, 氣海) | Heel | Death |
| Groin (Organ, 下陰) | Heel | Death |

Locations of exposed cavities when using kicking techniques in heel kick.

## 24. Step Forward and Strike Down with the Fist (Jin Bu Zai Chui, 進步栽捶)

### Movements

First, turn your body to your right while covering with your left arm to your right.

Next, step your left leg forward, and repel with your left arm to your left and down while punching your right fist downward.

### Analysis:

Both of your hands are used to intercept the lower punch or kick. Naturally, your right fist is for attack.

## Qin Na

### Technique #1. Two Children Worship the Buddha (Shuang Tong Bai Fo, 雙童拜佛)

Shuang tong bai fo is a technique that uses the movements of the step forward and strike down with the fist posture.

Situation: Your opponent punches your lower body with his left fist. Immediately use your left arm to neutralize his attack to your left.

Next, step your right leg behind his right leg, and hook his left arm upward while inserting your right arm under his left armpit and reaching his abdomen area.

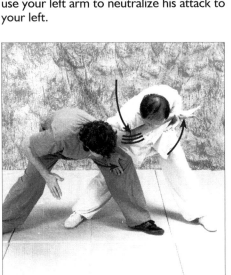

Then pull his left arm backward while pressing your right shoulder against his left shoulder, and push his left thigh with your left hand.

Finally, use this leverage to circle him down to the ground.

## Cavity Press or Strike:

Once you have used your left arm to clear his attack, you may use your right fist to attack the lower section of his body.

| Cavity name | Hand form(s) | Possible results |
| --- | --- | --- |
| Qimen (Li-14, 期門) | Fist | Seal the breath and rupture the liver |
| Riyue (GB-24, 日月) | Fist | Seal the breath and rupture the liver |
| Zhongwan (Co-12, 中脘) | Fist | Seal the breath and vomiting |
| Qihai (Co-6, 氣海) | Fist | Death |
| Groin (Organ, 下陰) | Fist | Death |

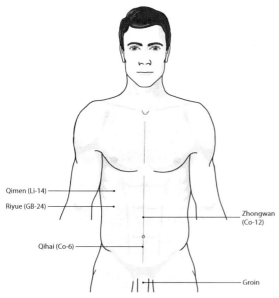

Locations of exposed cavities when using striking techniques in step forward and strike down.

## 25. Strike the Tiger (Da Hu Shi, 打虎勢)

### Movements

First, move your right arm upward and to your right while shifting your body forward into bow and arrow stance.

Next, move your left arm under your right arm and extend it forward while withdrawing your right hand back to the right side of your waist.

### Analysis:

Your right arm's upward movement is for interception. Then take this opportunity to grab his wrist with your left hand. Finally, pull him down with your left hand while using your right hand to strike.

Finally, squat down into the taming the tiger stance while pulling your left arm back to your left, and strike with your right hand in a circular motion.

## Qin Na

### Technique #1. The Arm Locks the Python's Neck (Bi Suo Mang Jing, 臂鎖蟒頸)

*Bi suo mang jing* is a technique that uses the movements of the strike the tiger posture.

Situation: Your opponent punches you with his left fist. First, use your right arm to intercept the punch.

Next, use your left hand to grab his left wrist.

Then reposition yourself behind him while circling your right arm around his neck.

Finally, pull his left arm back while locking his neck with your right arm.

## Cavity Press or Strike:

This technique aims the attack on the side or the back of your opponent's body.

| Cavity name | Hand form(s) | Possible results |
| --- | --- | --- |
| Shaohai (H-3, 少海) | Fingers (left) | Cause numbness |
| Quchi (LI-11, 曲池) | Fingers (left) | Cause numbness |
| Neiguan (P-6, 內關) | Fingers (left) | Cause numbness or fainting |
| Naohu (Gv-17, 腦戶) | Fist | Fainting, shock the brain |
| Tianzong (SI-11, 天宗) | Phoenix eye fist | Numbness |
| Lingtai (Gv-10, 靈台) | Fist | Death |

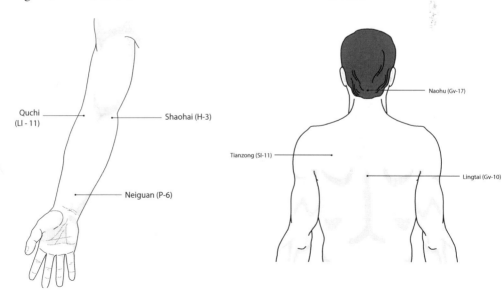

Locations of exposed cavities when using grabbing techniques in strike the tiger.

Locations of exposed cavities when using striking techniques in strike the tiger.

## 26. Two Winds Pass Through the Ears (Shuang Feng Guan Er, 雙風貫耳)

### Movements

First, move your right leg back and stand in false stance while lowering both of your arms in front of your chest.

Then circle both of your arms upward toward the center.

### Analysis:

You move your right leg backward so you can yield your body backward easily. Both of your arms' downward motion is to protect or to seal the attack to your chest. Your right leg's false stance can be used to kick anytime, since there is no weight on it. Finally, the arms' circling is to strike the opponent.

## Qin Na

### Technique #1. Force the Bow (Qiang Po Ju Gong, 強迫鞠躬)

Qiang po ju gong is a technique that uses the movements of the two winds pass through the ears posture.

Situation: Your opponent attacks you with his right fist. Immediately use your right hand to intercept the punch while stepping backward to yield.

Next, step your left leg behind him, and circle your right hand around his right arm while inserting your left arm under his left arm.

Finally, use both of your hands to press the upper back of his head downward to lock his neck.

## Cavity Press or Strike:

Neutralize your opponent's attack, either by pressing it downward or by repelling to the side.

Immediately attack the cavities on his head and neck.

| Cavity name | Hand form(s) | Possible results |
|---|---|---|
| Yifeng (TB-17, 翳風) | Thumb tip | Seal the artery |
| Futu (LI-18, 伏兔) | Thumb tip | Seal the artery |
| Taiyang (M-HN-9, 太陽) | Phoenix eye fist | Death (rupture the artery) |
| Ermen (TB-21, 耳門) | Knuckle of thumb | Fainting |
| Jiache (S-6, 頰車) | Back of fist | Fainting |

Taiyang (M-HN-9)

Ermen (TB-21)

Yifeng (TB-17)

Jiache (S-6)

Futu (LI-18)

Location of exposed cavities when using striking techniques in two winds pass through the ears.

## 27. Wild Horses Shear the Mane (Ye Ma Fen Zong, 野馬分鬃)

### Movements

First, turn your body to your left, withdraw your right leg so that it is next to your left leg, and move your left arm upward and then sideways while lowering your right arm.

Next, step your right leg forward while spreading your arms diagonally.

### Analysis:

This is the movement of rend (lie). Your right leg withdrawing is yielding to the opponent's attack. Your left hand's upward and sideways movement is for intercepting and neutralizing. The spreading action is for an attack.

## Qin Na

### Technique #1. Wild Horses Shear the Mane (Ye Ma Fen Zong, 野馬分鬃)

Ye ma fen zong is a technique that uses the movements of the wild horses shear the mane posture.

Situation: Your opponent punches you with his right fist. Immediately withdraw your right leg back while using your left forearm to intercept and neutralize the attack.

Then step your right leg in while using your right forearm to lock the tendons of your opponent's post-arm.

## Cavity Press or Strike:

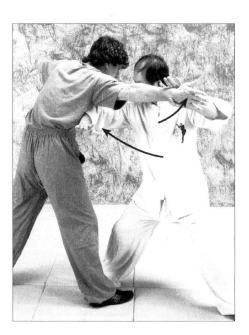

Once you have used your left arm to clear his attack, you have exposed the right side of his body to your attack. You can then use your fist or even elbow to attack.

| Cavity name | Hand form(s) | Possible results |
|---|---|---|
| Qimen (Li-14, 期門) | Phoenix eye fist or elbow | Seal the breath and rupture the liver |
| Riyue (GB-24, 日月) | Phoenix eye fist or elbow | Seal the breath and rupture the liver |

Qimen (Li-14)

Riyue (GB-24)

Locations of exposed cavities when using striking techniques in wild horses shear the mane.

## 28. Fair Lady Weaves with Shuttle (Yu Niu Chuan Suo, 玉女穿梭)

### Movements

First, lower your left arm while circling your left hand to the left of your waist.

Then shift your weight to your right and enter a bow and arrow stance while raising your right arm and starting to push your left hand forward.

## Analysis:

Your right arm is used to neutralize the opponent's power upward and to the side. Therefore, it is a wardoff (peng). Your left hand's palm attack is a press forward (*an*, 按).

Finally, turn your body to your right while rotating your right arm to your right and pushing your left palm forward.

## Qin Na

### Technique #1. Forward Upward Turning (Qian Shang Fan, 前上翻)

Qian shang fan is a technique that uses the movements of the fair lady weaves with shuttle posture.

Situation: Your opponent is punching you with his right fist. Immediately use your right forearm to intercept and neutralize his attack upward and to your right while using your left hand to seal his right elbow.

Next, step your right leg behind his right leg while pressing his elbow inward and pushing his wrist forward to make it bend and lock it.

Finally, let your left hand take over the control of his wrist and arm while using your right hand to push the upper back of his head forward.

## Cavity Press or Strike:

Once you have used your right arm to intercept and neutralize your opponent's power upward and to the side, you have exposed the area under his armpit to your attack. In this case, you may use the palm to strike his lower ribs, phoenix eye fist to attack the nerves between his ribs, or fingers to attack his cavity.

| Cavity name | Hand form(s) | Possible results |
|---|---|---|
| Jiquan (H-1, 極泉) | Sword secret | Cause a heart attack |

Jiquan
(H-1)

Location of exposed cavity when using striking techniques in fair lady weaves with shuttle.

## 29. Lower the Snake Body (She Shen Xia Shi, 蛇身下勢)

### Movements

Begin from the end of the single whip posture.

First, move your left hand toward you with the palm facing you while squatting on your right leg. Then extend your left arm out along the inner side of your left leg.

## Analysis:

Although in the practice you squat down very low to train your knees' strength, in actual application you only squat down enough to yield to the oncoming attack. The key application of this posture is the left arm's coiling (chan, 纏).

## Qin Na

### Technique #1: Reverse Elbow Wrap (Fan Chan Zhou, 反纏肘)

Fan chan zhou is a technique that uses the movements of the lower the snake body posture.

Situation: Your opponent attacks you with his right fist. Immediately squat down and sit backward while using your left forearm to intercept and neutralize the attack to your right.

Next, coil your left hand around his right arm until it reaches his post-arm.

Finally, use the leverage generated from your left hand and elbow to press him down to the ground.

## Cavity Press or Strike:

Your left hand's coiling movement can lead and neutralize your opponent's attack to his right. You can use this opportunity and immediately attack the right side of his body with your right hand.

| Cavity name | Hand form(s) | Possible results |
| --- | --- | --- |
| Ruzhong (S-17, 乳中) | Palm | Seal the breath |
| Rugen (S-18, 乳根) | Palm | Seal the breath |
| Qimen (Li-14, 期門) | Fist or phoenix eye fist | Seal the breath and rupture the liver |
| Riyue (GB-24, 日月) | Fist or phoenix eye fist | Seal the breath and rupture the liver |

Ruzhong (S-17)
Rugen (S-18)
Qimen (Li-14)
Riyue (GB-24)

Locations of exposed cavities when using striking techniques in lower the snake body.

## 30. Golden Rooster Stands on One Leg (Jin Ji Du Li, 金雞獨立)

### Movements

First, turn your body to the left while starting to raise your right arm.

Then raise your right knee while lifting your right arm until the palm is as high as your face.

### Analysis:

Your left arm can be used to repel the oncoming attack, and the right hand and the knee are used to attack.

## Qin Na

### Technique #1. Golden Rooster Locks the Arm (Jin Ji Suo Bi, 金雞鎖臂)

*Jin ji suo bi* is a technique that uses the movements of the golden rooster stands on one leg posture. In fact, this qin na is used only to lock your opponent's arm, which can therefore create an opportunity for your leg's attack.

Situation: Your have a chance to grab your opponent's left wrist with your left hand. Immediately insert your right forearm behind his post-arm.

Next, using the leverage of your left hand and right arm, you may lock your opponent's right arm.

This technique can lock your opponent's right arm for only a short time. It is not practical to lock it for a long time, since his left hand is able to reach you easily. Therefore, right after your locking, you should immediately strike his groin with your right knee.

## Cavity Press or Strike:

Right after your left hand's neutralization, you may use your right hand to attack his upper body while using your right knee to attack his lower body.

| Cavity name | Hand form(s) | Possible results |
|---|---|---|
| Throat | Fingers' grabbing | Seal the breath |
| Tiantu (Co-22, 天突) | Thumb | Seal the breath |
| Qihai (Co-6, 氣海) | Knee | Death |
| Groin (Organ, 下陰) | Knee | Death |

Tiantu (Co-22)

Qihai (Co-6)

Locations of exposed cavities when using grabbing, striking, or kicking techniques in golden rooster stands on one leg.

### 31. White Snake Turns Body and Spits Poison (Bai She Tu Xin, 白蛇吐信)

**Movements**

Begin from the end of the fan back posture.

Turn your body to your right while lowering your right arm.

**Analysis:**

Normally, this posture is used against the opponent's attack from behind. Your right arm is used to repel the attack while the left hand is used to attack his face with great speed, just like a snake spitting poison from its mouth.

Then shift your weight to your right leg and enter a bow and arrow stance while repelling with your right arm to your right and striking your left palm forward.

## Qin Na

### Technique #1. Lock the Arm and Push the Neck (Suo Bi Tui Jing, 鎖臂推頸)

*Suo bi tui jing* is a technique that uses the movements of the white snake turns body and spits poison: lock arm and push neck posture.

Situation: Your opponent punches your lower body. Use your right forearm to repel his attack to your right.

Next, step your left leg behind his right leg while hooking his right arm up with your right arm and extending your left arm to lock his neck. If you wish to take him down, simply sweep your left leg forward while pressing his neck backward.

### Cavity Press or Strike:

Your right arm is used to repel the attack to the side, while your left hand catches the opportunity to attack.

| Cavity name | Hand form(s) | Possible results |
| --- | --- | --- |
| Eyes | Fingers | Blinding |
| Shangen (M-HN-4, 山根) | Fist | Fainting, nose bleeding |
| Renzhong (Gv-26, 人中) | Fist | Fainting |

Shangen
(M-HN-4)

Renzhong
(Gv-26)

Locations of exposed cavities when using striking techniques
in white snake turns body and spits poison.

## 32. Cross Hands (Shi Zi Shou, 十字手)

### Movements

Begin from the end of the stand high to search out the horse posture.

Step your left leg forward and enter a bow and arrow stance while covering down with your right arm and extending your left arm upward and forward.

## Analysis:

Your right arm's covering is used to neutralize the attack downward, which can therefore expose the opponent's face to your attack.

## Qin Na

### Technique #1. Daoist Greets with Hands (Dao Zi Zuo Ji, 道子作揖)

Dao zi zuo ji is a technique that uses the movements of the cross hands posture. This technique uses the arm's crossing action to lock the opponent's arm.

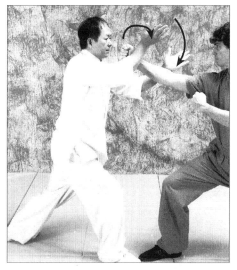

Situation: Your opponent attacks you with his right hand. Immediately use your right hand to intercept his right forearm, while using your left hand to push his right elbow to your right.

Then step your left leg behind his right leg and use both of your hands to rotate his right arm and lock it in place.

## Cavity Press or Strike:

Your right hand is used to neutralize the attack to your left and then downward.

After your neutralization, you may immediately attack your opponent's face with your left hand. You may use your right fist to attack his right lower rib area immediately following your left hand's face attack.

| Cavity name | Hand form(s) | Possible results |
| --- | --- | --- |
| Eyes | Fingers | Blinding |
| Shangen (M-HN-4, 山根) | Fist | Fainting, nose bleeding |
| Renzhong (Gv-26, 人中) | Fist | Fainting |
| Throat | Fingers' grabbing | Seal the breath |
| Tiantu (Co-22, 天突) | Thumb | Seal the breath |

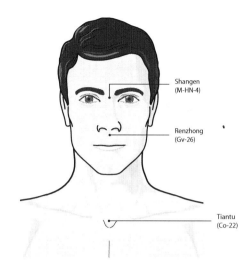

Shangen
(M-HN-4)

Renzhong
(Gv-26)

Tiantu
(Co-22)

Locations of exposed cavities when using grabbing or striking techniques in cross hands.

## 33. The Word "Ten" Leg (Shi Zi Tui, 十字腿)

### Movements

First, cross both of your arms in front of your chest while moving your right leg back.

Next, open both of your arms and use your right leg to kick.

### Analysis:

This posture is named "the word 'ten' leg posture" because it is shaped like the Chinese for "ten." Both of your arms are used to intercept the chest's attack or grab, and the leg is used to kick.

## Qin Na

### Technique #1. The Word "Ten" Pressing Leg (Shi Zi Ding Tui, 十字頂腿)

*Shi zi ding tui* is a technique that uses the movements of the word "ten" leg posture.

Situation: Your opponent punches your chest with his right fist. Immediately use your right forearm to intercept the attack and grab his wrist.

Next, pull his right wrist down; this will offer your opponent a chance to attack you with his left hand. In this situation, immediately use your left hand to intercept the punch and grab his left wrist.

Then reposition yourself to his back while pulling both of his arms down behind him.

Finally, use your right leg to press his sacrum forward to lock him in place.

## Cavity Press or Strike:

Once you have used both of your hands to grab both of his wrists, you may kick the lower section of his body with your right leg.

This technique can also be used against a grabbing or an attack from behind.

In this case, first turn your body and use your right hand to grab his wrist.

Then immediately kick his right lower rib area with your right leg.

| Cavity name | Hand form(s) | Possible results |
|---|---|---|
| Riyue (GB-24, 日月) | Heel | Seal the breath and rupture the liver |
| Zhongwan (Co-12, 中脘) | Heel | Seal the breath and vomiting |
| Qihai (Co-6, 氣海) | Heel | Death |
| Groin (Organ, 下陰) | Heel or toes | Death |

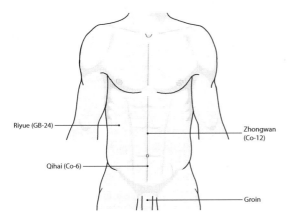

Locations of exposed cavities when using kicking techniques in the word "ten" leg posture.

## 34. Step Forward to Seven Stars (Shang Bu Qi Xing, 上步七星)

### Movements

Begin from the end of the lower the snake body posture.

Shift your weight to your left leg while raising your left arm.

**Analysis:**

Your right arm is used to deflect the opponent's power upward; it can also be extended forward either for punching or locking his elbow. Naturally, your right leg can be used for kicking.

Then step your right leg forward into false stance while punching your right fist forward.

**Qin Na**

### Technique #1. Seven Stars to Lock the Throat (Qi Xing Suo Hou, 七星鎖喉)

*Qi xing suo hou* is a technique that uses the movements of the step forward to seven stars posture.

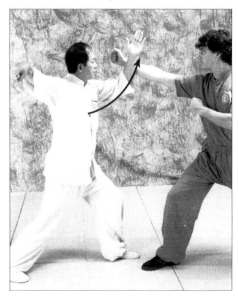

Situation: Your opponent attacks you with his right fist. First, use your left forearm to repel his punch.

Next, step your right leg forward, pushing his right forearm forward while using your right forearm to pull in his elbow.

Finally, grab his throat with your right hand while still locking his right arm.

## Cavity Press or Strike:

Once you have used your left arm to clear his attack, you may use your right fist to attack the right side of his body.

| Cavity name | Hand form(s) | Possible results |
| --- | --- | --- |
| Ruzhong (S-17, 乳中) | Fist | Seal the breath |
| Rugen (S-18, 乳根) | Fist | Seal the breath |
| Qimen (Li-14, 期門) | Fist | Seal the breath and rupture the liver |
| Riyue (GB-24, 日月) | Fist | Seal the breath and rupture the liver |
| Qihai (Co-6, 氣海) | Heel | Death |
| Groin (Organ, 下陰) | Toes | Death |

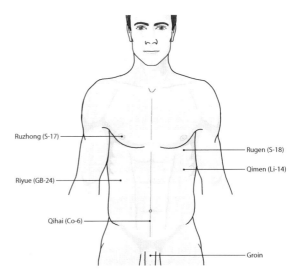

Locations of exposed cavities when using striking or kicking techniques in step forward to seven stars.

## 35. Step Back to Ride the Tiger (Tui Bu Kua Hu, 退步跨虎)

## Movements

Begin from the end of the step forward to seven stars posture.

Step your right leg backward while spreading your arms diagonally.

## Analysis:

Both of your arms are used to spread out the oncoming attack while your left leg is ready for kicking.

## Qin Na

No qin na available.

## Cavity Press or Strike:

Use both of your arms to repel your opponent's attack outward.

You will have exposed the center area of his body for your kicking.

| Cavity name | Hand form(s) | Possible results |
|---|---|---|
| Zhongwan (Co-12, 中脘) | Heel | Seal the breath and vomiting |
| Qihai (Co-6, 氣海) | Heel | Death |
| Groin (Organ, 下陰) | Heel or toes | Death |

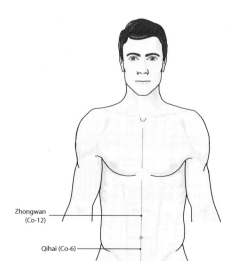

Locations of exposed cavities when using kicking techniques in step back to ride the tiger.

## 36. Step Forward to Sweep Lotus (Shang Bu Bai Lian, 上步擺蓮)

**Movements**

First, turn your body to your left while crossing both of your arms in front of your chest.

Then spread your arms outward while lifting your knee upward.

### Analysis:

If your chest has been grabbed by both of your opponent's hands, you can use both of your arms to repel his grabbing outward and then grab his arms or shoulder area. In this situation, he will not be able to escape, and this will allow you to strike him with your right knee.

## Qin Na

### Technique #1. Two Hands Push the Chest (Shuang Shou Tui Xiong, 雙手推胸)

*Shuang shou tui xiong* is a technique that uses the movements of the step forward to sweep lotus posture.

Situation: Both of your opponent's hands are grabbing your upper chest. Immediately use both of your arms to repel his grabbing.

Next, coil both of your arms to the outside of both of his arms, and then push both of your hands toward his chest to lock his arms.

## Cavity Press or Strike:

Once you have locked both of his arms, you may use your right knee to strike the lower section of his body.

| Cavity name | Hand form(s) | Possible results |
|---|---|---|
| Qihai (Co-6, 氣海) | Knee | Death |
| Groin (Organ, 下陰) | Knee | Death |

Qihai (Co-6)

Locations of exposed cavities when using kicking techniques in step forward to sweep lotus.

### 37. Draw the Bow and Shoot the Tiger (Wan Gong She Hu, 彎弓射虎)

**Movements**

First, step your left leg backward while scooping your right arm upward.

Then raise your right arm up to your right while punching your left fist forward.

## Analysis:

Your backward stepping is to yield to the oncoming power, and your right arm's upward movement is for intercepting and neutralizing. Naturally, your left fist's forward action is for an attack.

## Qin Na

### Technique #1. Roast Peking Duck (Bei Ping Kao Ya, 北平烤鴨)

Bei Ping kao ya is a technique that uses the movements of the draw the bow and shoot the tiger posture.

Situation: Your opponent uses his right hand to grab or punch your upper chest. Immediately use your right forearm to intercept the attack and then grab his hand while inserting your left arm under his right arm until it reaches his neck.

Next, twist his arm counterclockwise until his right palm faces upward. Then pull his arm down while lifting your left elbow to lock his right arm.

**Technique #2. Lock the Arm and Push the Neck (Suo Bi Tui Jing, 鎖臂推頸)**

Suo bi tui jing is a technique that uses the movements of the draw the bow and shoot the tiger posture.

Situation: Your opponent punches your chest with his right fist. Immediately use your right forearm to intercept and then grab his right wrist while using your left forearm to push his right elbow to keep his arm bent.

Then step your left leg behind his right leg, and pull his right arm against your chest while extending your left arm to his neck and lock him there.

**Technique #3. Old Man Carries the Fish on His Back (Lao Han Bei Yu, 老漢背魚)**

Lao han bei yu is a technique that uses the movements of the draw the bow and shoot the tiger posture.

Situation: Your opponent punches your chest with his right fist. Immediately use your right forearm to intercept and then grab his right wrist while using your left forearm to push his right elbow to keep his arm bent.

Immediately step your left leg behind his right leg, turn your body to your right, and then pull his arm downward to lock his right arm.

**Cavity Press or Strike:**

Once you have used your right arm to neutralize the oncoming attack, you will have exposed the area under his armpit to your attack.

| Cavity name | Hand form(s) | Possible results |
| --- | --- | --- |
| Jiquan (H-1, 極泉) | Sword secret | Cause a heart attack |
| Yuanye (GB-22, 淵腋) | Phoenix eye fist | Seal the breath |
| Dabao (Sp-21, 大包) | Phoenix eye fist | Seal the breath |

Jiquan (H-1)

Yuanye (GB-22)

Dabao (Sp-21)

Locations of exposed cavities when using striking techniques in draw the bow and shoot the tiger.

# Chapter 6: Qin Na in Taiji Pushing Hands

## 6-1. Introduction

We know that taijiquan is a martial art that was created and designed for combat. Furthermore, we also know that in order to reach the final goal of fighting capability in taijiquan, a taiji practitioner must follow the designed training steps to build up the required fighting skills. Qin na is only one of the four categories of fighting techniques.

Traditionally, when you start taijiquan practice, you will first be taught some simple taiji qigong and breathing techniques. These are the first few steps that can lead you to the entrance of understanding and feeling the qi circulation in your body. Next, you will learn how to use your mind to lead the qi (*yi yi yin qi*, 以意引氣). Only when you understand and are able to feel the qi and know how to use your mind to lead the qi, will you have built up a firm foundation of the internal side of taijiquan practice. Taiji qigong should be practiced at all times in taijiquan practice. It is not merely trained at the beginner stage. The more advanced levels of taijiquan can be reached only through deeper qigong practice.

Often, when you start your taiji qigong, you will also be taught some basic relaxation movements and fundamental stances. After you have become familiar with the basic relaxation movements, the taijiquan sequence will be taught. Although there are only thirty-seven postures in the traditional Yang Style Taijiquan 105-movement routine, there are more than 250 martial applications, including striking, kicking, wrestling, and qin na, which can be derived from the thirty-seven postures. Traditionally, the secrets of these martial techniques must be revealed by a master. Only when you have learned the martial applications can every taijiquan movement exhibit its essence, root, and meaning. Otherwise, the movements will only be some relaxation exercises. If taijiquan becomes merely a type of relaxation exercise, then anybody will be able to create a style, and the movements of the style will be classified only as relaxation/health qigong instead of taijiquan.

In order to help you understand the martial applications of taijiquan, normally taiji pushing hands practice is introduced first. From pushing hands practice, you will learn how to feel the opponent's jing (martial power) and qi. From this feeling (i.e., listening jing, 聽勁), you will learn how to stick and adhere your body to your opponent's body. Sticking and adhering allows you to direct and neutralize your opponent's attacking power into emptiness. Normally, it will take many years of pushing hands training to reach a high level of skill. Only after you are able to reach a high level of pushing hands will your striking by hands and kicking by legs be effective, since your opponent will always be under your control.

Naturally, in order to reach this goal, your body must be soft, especially your spine and waist. In addition, your qi must be strong and must circulate smoothly and freely. All of these are also basic requirements for health. Therefore, taiji pushing hands practice is one of the most effective ways of maintaining and improving your health. Also, through practice, both qi and ideas can be exchanged between you and your partner. This can also establish good qi feelings and friendship.

From the above, you can see that pushing hands practice is actually a necessary step to reaching the final goal of taiji fighting practice. Since in taijiquan pushing hands you must stick and adhere your hands or even your body to your opponent's, the range is close and mutual contact is constantly maintained. Qin na is the most efficient and effective technique for placing your opponent into a controlled situation.

This chapter will summarize and review some of the qin na techniques that can be used in pushing hands situations. Naturally, since most taiji pushing hands techniques are derived from the eight basic, technical moving patterns—peng, lu, ji, *an*, cai, lie, zhou, and kao—it is not surprising to see that many of the qin na techniques in this chapter are refinements of those techniques that have already been introduced in chapters 3 and 4. Part of your training is learning the qin na techniques from chapters 3 and 4, and then applying them to taiji pushing hands by yourself. Hopefully we have established a guideline and understanding of how qin na can be adopted in taiji pushing hands so your personal training can progress.

Naturally, since there are so many qin na techniques available, you will discover that some of the techniques introduced in this chapter were not discussed earlier. If you are interested in learning more about the internal aspects of taiji qigong practice, you may refer to the book *Tai Chi Qigong*, published by YMAA. In addition, if you are interested in learning more about qin na techniques, you may refer to the books *Analysis of Shaolin Chin Na* and *Comprehensive Applications of Shaolin Chin Na*, published by YMAA.

## 6-2. Qin Na in Taiji Pushing Hands

In taiji pushing hands, it is desirable to control your opponent's joints as much as possible. The reason for this is simply because when the joints are controlled, the mobility of your opponent's arms will be restricted. Therefore, in this section, we will divide the sample qin na techniques that can be used in pushing hands into three categories: qin na against hands on your wrist or forearm, qin na against hands on your elbow joints, and qin na against hands on your shoulder joints.

## I. Against Hands on Wrist Joints or Forearms

### Technique #1. Small Wrap Finger (Xiao Chan Zhi, 小纏指)

*Xiao chan zhi* is a technique that uses qin na against hands on your wrist or forearm.

Situation: Your opponent's right hand is on your right wrist.

Immediately reposition yourself to his right side while neutralizing his pressing to your right. As you do this, also use your left hand to pull his pinkie toward your right wrist while wrapping your right hand around his wrist.

Finally, press his wrist down with your right hand while pulling his pinkie strongly toward your right wrist.

To control him, his elbow should be lower than his wrist; otherwise. he will be able to turn his body counterclockwise to release the control, and the technique will not be effective.

## Technique #2. Small Wrap Hand (Xiao Chan Shou, 小纏手)

Xiao chan shou is a technique that uses qin na against hands on your wrist or forearm. This technique is very similar to the last one. The only difference is that instead of controlling the pinkie, you pull his index finger toward your wrist.

Situation: Your opponent's right hand is on your right wrist.

Immediately turn your body to your right to neutralize the press while using your left hand to pull his index finger toward your right wrist and wrapping your right hand around his right wrist.

Then reposition yourself to his right side while pressing your right hand down against his right wrist.

To make the control effective, his elbow should be lower than his wrist.

## Technique #3. Back Wrap Hand (Fan Chan Shou, 反纏手)

*Fan chan shou* is a technique that uses qin na against hands on your wrist or forearm.

Situation: Your opponent's right hand is on your right wrist. Turn your body to your right to neutralize his pressing.

Next, use your left hand to grab his right fingers.

Then use both hands to circle his arm downward.

Follow with an upward circle to lock his wrist.

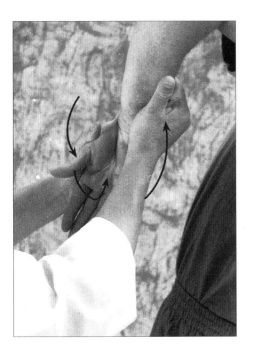

To make the technique most effective, you should use your left hand to twist his wrist as much as possible, while using your right hand to lock his forearm, and generate good leverage for your left hand's twisting.

## Technique #4. Large Wrap Hand (Da Chan Shou, 大纏手)

Da chan shou is a technique that uses qin na against hands on your wrist or forearm.

Situation: Your opponent presses your right wrist with his right hand. Immediately turn your body to your right to neutralize the pressing.

Next, reposition yourself to his right side while circling your left hand under his right arm until it reaches his right index finger, and wrap your right hand around his right wrist.

Finally, press his wrist down while pushing his index finger toward your right wrist.

## Technique #5. Upward Elbow Wrap (Shang Chan Zhou, 上纏肘)

Shang chan zhou is a technique that uses qin na against hands on your wrist or forearm.

Situation: Your opponent's right hand is on your right wrist. Immediately turn your body to your right to neutralize the pressing or grabbing while using your left hand to grab his right hand.

Next, circle his arm upward with both of your hands.

Then reposition yourself to his right side while twisting his wrist with your left hand and lifting his elbow with your right hand to lock him up.

You may also lock his right arm with your right hand and stomach area while using your left forearm to push his neck away to generate pain.

### Technique #6. Small Elbow Wrap (Xiao Chan Zhou, 小纏肘)

Xiao chan zhou is a technique that uses qin na against hands on your wrist or forearm.

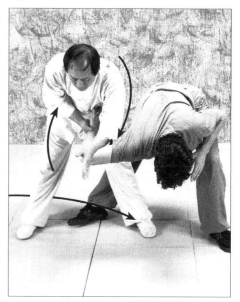

Situation: Your opponent's right hand is pressing on your right wrist. In order to neutralize your opponent, turn your body to your right.

Next, step your left leg to the front of his right leg, and grab his right wrist with your right hand while pressing his elbow downward with your left forearm.

Finally, sweep your left leg backward while using the leverage generated from both of your hands to circle him down to the ground.

## Technique #7. Reverse Elbow Wrap (Fan Chan Zhou, 反纏肘)

Fan chan zhou is a technique that uses qin na against hands on your wrist or forearm.

Situation: Your opponent's right hand is pressing on your right wrist. Turn your body to your right to neutralize him.

Next, reposition yourself to his right side, and grab his right wrist with your right hand while coiling your left hand around his arm until it reaches his post-arm near the elbow.

Finally, use the leverage generated from your left hand and elbow to circle him down to the ground.

### Technique #8. Upward Elbow Press (Shang Ya Zhou, 上壓肘)

*Shang ya zhou* is a technique that uses qin na against hands on your wrist or forearm.

Situation: Your opponent's right hand is on your right wrist. Immediately turn your body to your right while placing your left hand on his right elbow.

Then reposition yourself to his right, circle your right hand and grab his right wrist, and press his right wrist down while using your left hand to push his right elbow upward.

## Technique #9. Daoist Greets with Hands (Dao Zi Zuo Ji, 道子作揖)

Dao zi zuo ji is a technique that uses qin na against hands on your wrist or forearm. This technique is very similar to shang ya zhou (upward elbow press). The only difference is that this technique can be used if your opponent keeps his arm straight, which can prevent you from locking his elbow as executed in shang ya zhou.

Situation: Your opponent's right hand is pressing or grabbing your right wrist. Turn your body to your right to neutralize his right hand pressing or grabbing while placing your left forearm on his elbow.

Then reposition yourself to his right side, circle your right hand to grab his right wrist, and pull it down while pushing his elbow upward to keep it bent. This will allow you to lock his right arm. To prevent him from turning his body, simply use your left shoulder to push his right shoulder. This will stop him from turning.

### Technique #10. Old Man Carries the Fish on His Back (Lao Han Bei Yu, 老漢背魚)

Lao han bei yu is a technique that uses qin na against hands on your wrist or forearm.

Situation: Your opponent is pressing or grabbing your right wrist. Immediately neutralize to your right.

Step your right leg behind him, and pull his right arm down while using your back to lock his arm in place. To make this control effective, your opponent's arm should be neither too straight nor too bent.

## Technique #11. Send the Devil to Heaven (Song Mo Shang Tian, 送魔上天)

Song mo shang tian is a technique that uses qin na against hands on your wrist or forearm.

Situation: Your opponent's right hand is on your right wrist, pulling your right arm to his right.

Immediately step your right leg to his right, moving your right arm up and to his right while using your left hand to grab his right hand.

Then step your left leg behind him and use your body's left turning momentum to lock him up.

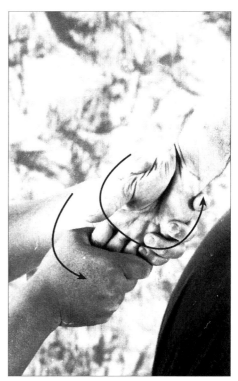

The most effective way to lock his arm is to use your left hand to twist his right wrist while using your right hand to grab his fingers and bend them downward.

## II. Against Hands on Elbow Joints

### Technique #1. Feudal Lord Lifts the Tripod (Ba Wang Tai Ding, 霸王抬鼎)

Ba wang tai ding is a technique that uses qin na against hands on your elbow joints.

Situation: Your opponent's left hand is adhering on your right elbow.

Immediately scoop your right arm upward while using your left hand to grab his left hand.

Next, twist his left wrist with your left hand while using your right hand to push his left elbow to keep it bent.

Finally, lift his left elbow with your right hand while twisting his left wrist continuously.

## Technique #2. Arm Wraps Around the Dragon's Neck (Bi Chan Long Jing, 臂纏龍頸)

Bi chan long jing is a technique that uses qin na against hands on your elbow joints.

Situation: Your opponent's left hand is adhering on your right elbow.

Immediately scoop your right arm upward while using your left hand to grab his left hand.

Next, lock his left arm on your stomach area while extending your right arm to his neck.

Finally, circle your right arm around his neck while continuing to lock his left arm.

## Technique #3. Crane Spreads Its Wings (Bai He Liang Chi, 白鶴亮翅)

Bai he liang chi is a technique that uses qin na against hands on your elbow joints.

(This technique is very similar to bi chan long jing.) Situation: Your opponent's left hand is on your right elbow. Immediately scoop your right arm upward while using your left hand to grab his left hand.

Next, twist his left wrist with your left hand while using your right hand to push his forearm.

Finally, expand your right arm on his neck while continuing to twist his wrist. This will provide you with good leverage for locking his arm.

## III. Against Hands on Shoulder Joints

### Technique #1. The Hero Shows Courtesy (Ying Xiong You Li, 英雄有禮)

Ying xiong you li is a technique that uses qin na against hands on your shoulder joints.

Situation: Your opponent's right hand is on your left shoulder. Immediately use your right hand to grab his right hand.

Next, circle your left arm over his forearm.

Reposition yourself and use the leverage generated from your left arm and right hand to lock his right wrist.

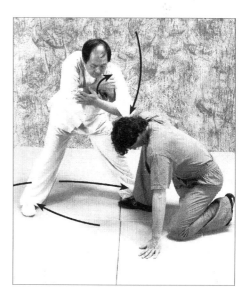

## Technique #2: Press Shoulder with Single Finger / Extending the Neck for Water (Yi Zhi Ding Jian / Yin Jing Qiu Shui, 一指頂肩 / 引頸求水)

Yi zhi ding jian / yin jing qiu shui is a technique that uses qin na against hands on your shoulder joints.

Situation: Your opponent's right hand is on your left shoulder. Immediately use your right hand to grab his right hand.

Next, free your left hand and place it on your opponent's right elbow.

Then reposition yourself to his right side while coiling your left hand around his right arm until it reaches his post-arm, and raise it upward to lock his arm.

Finally, use your right index finger to press his jianneiling cavity to increase the pain.

Alternatively, you may use your hand to press his chin upward to generate leverage for locking.

## Technique #3. Old Man Promoted to General (Lao Han Bai Jiang, 老漢拜將)

Lao han bai jiang is a technique that uses qin na against hands on your shoulder joints.

Situation: Your opponent's right hand is on your left shoulder.

Use your right hand to grab his right hand while circling your left arm over his right arm.

Next, place his right elbow under your left armpit while lifting his wrist upward.

Finally, use the leverage generated from both of your hands and left shoulder to press him down to the ground.

Remember, this chapter offers you only some of the qin na applications. You should study chapters 3 and 4 carefully and apply them to your pushing hands. The best method of learning is practicing with a partner.

# Chapter 7: Conclusion

Although this book offers you only some of my personal knowledge about the possible qin na applications in Yang Style Taijiquan, it can provide you with an idea and correct concept of how qin na can be applied in taijiquan. I hope that from this book you are inspired and encouraged to get involved in more study and research into the martial applications of taijiquan. Naturally, if you are already an expert in any style of taijiquan and have also mastered the martial applications of the style, you should not hesitate to write them down, offer seminars, and introduce them to taijiquan society. Only then can this art remain alive and develop continuously.

To help you achieve an in-depth understanding of taijiquan, both in theory and application, you may refer to the books *Tai Chi Theory and Martial Power* and *Tai Chi Chuan Martial Applications*. However, if you would like to know more about the internal cultivation of qi, and how qi is applied in taijiquan, then you should read *Tai Chi Qigong*.

If this book has inspired you to learn more about qin na, then you may refer to *Analysis of Shaolin Chin Na* and *Comprehensive Applications of Shaolin Chin Na*. All of these books are available from YMAA.

# Acknowledgements

### First Edition (1995)

Thanks to Tim Comrie for his photography, Jerry Leake for design and layout, and James B. Philips for the cover drawing. Thanks also to Yang, Mei-Ling, Ramel Rones, and Craig McConnell for general help, to Ray Ahles, David W. Grantham, Andrew Murray, Jeffrey Pratt, David Ripianzi, and many other YMAA members for proofing the manuscript and for contributing many valuable suggestions and discussions. Special thanks to James O'Leary for his editing. And a very special thanks to Liang Dexing (Jeffrey D. S. Liang) for his beautiful calligraphy on the front pages of this volume.

### Second Edition (2014)

The publisher wishes to thank Axie Breen for the cover design, Dolores Sparrow for copyediting and indexing, T. G. LaFredo for copyediting, Leslie Takao for caption editing, and Sara Scanlon for proofreading.

# Appendix A

## Names of Qin Na Techniques

Arm Locks the Python's Neck (Bi Suo Mang Jing, 臂鎖蟒頸)

Arm Rolls Back the Enemy's Elbow (Bi Lu Di Zhou, 臂攄敵肘)

Arm Wards Off the Enemy's Leg (Bi Peng Di Tui, 臂掤敵腿)

Arm Wraps Around the Dragon's Neck (Bi Chan Long Jing, 臂纏龍頸)

Back Wrap Hand (Fan Chan Shou, 反纏手)

Backward Upward Turning (Hou Shang Fan, 後上翻)

Both Hands Seize the Murderer (Shuang Shou Qin Xiong, 雙手擒凶)

Both Hands Twist the Neck (Shuang Shou Niu Jing, 雙手扭頸)

Butterfly Bores Through the flowers (Hu Die Chuan Hua, 蝴蝶穿花)

Carry a Pole on the Shoulder (Jian Tiao Bian Dan, 肩挑扁擔)

Child Worships the Buddha (Tong Zi Bai Fo, 童子拜佛)

Cloud Hands to Lock the Elbow (Yun Shou Jia Zhou, 雲手架肘)

Crane Spreads Its Wings (Bai He Liang Chi, 白鶴亮翅)

Daoist Greets with Hands (Dao Zi Zuo Ji, 道子作揖)

Diagonal Flying (Xie Fei Shi, 斜飛式)

Diagonal Flying to Support the Arm (Xie Fei Cheng Bi, 斜飛撐臂)

Double Hands Push the Mountain (Shuang Shou Tui Shan, 雙手推山)

Embrace Tiger and Return to the Mountain (Bao Hu Gui Shan, 抱虎歸山)

Extending the Neck for Water (Yin Jing Qiu Shui, 引頸求水)

Fair Lady Picks the Peach (Xian Niu Zhai Tao, 仙女摘桃)

Feudal Lord Lifts the Tripod (Ba Wang Tai Ding, 霸王抬鼎)

Feudal Lord Pushes the Caldron (Ba Wang Tui Ding, 霸王推鼎)

Force the Bow (Qiang Po Jiu Gong, 強迫鞠躬)

Forcarm Wardoff thc Encmy's Elbow (Bi Pcng Di Zhou, 臂掤敵肘)

Forgive Me for Not Going with You (Shu Bu Tong Xing, 恕不同行)

Forward Upward Turning (Qian Shang Fan, 前上翻)

Golden Rooster Locks the Arm (Jin Ji Suo Bi, 金雞鎖臂)

Grasp Sparrow's Tail (Lan Qiu Wei, 攬雀尾)

Hand Bends the Pine Branch (Shou Ban Song Zhi, 手扳松枝)

Hands Grab Double Cavities (Shou Kou Shuang Xue, 手扣雙穴)

Hands Hold a Panda (Shou Bao Wan Xiong, 手抱浣熊)

Heaven King Supports the Pagoda (Tian Wang Tuo Ta, 天王托塔)

Hero Shows Courtesy (Ying Xiong You Li, 英雄有禮)

Knee Presses the Enemy's Leg (Xi Ding Di Tui, 膝頂敵腿)

Large Ape Bends the Branch (Da Yuan Pan Zhi, 大猿攀枝)

Large Elbow Wrap (Da Chan Zhou, 大纏肘)

Large Python Coils the Neck (Da Mang Chan Jing, 大蟒纏頸)

Large Rollback (Da Lu, 大擺)

Large Wrap Hand (Da Chan Shou, 大纏手)

Lead the Snake to Enter the Cave (Yin She Ru Dong, 引蛇入洞)

Left Right Cross Elbow (Zuo You Jiao Zhou, 左右交肘)

Leg Twists the Enemy's Leg (Tui Ban Di Tui, 腿絆敵腿)

Lock the Arm and Push the Neck (Suo Bi Tui Jing, 鎖臂推頸)

Low Outward Wrist Press (Xia Wai Ya Wan, 下外壓腕)

Old Man Carries the Fish on His Back (Lao Han Bei Yu, 老漢背魚)

Old Man Promoted to General (Lao Han Bai Jiang, 老漢拜將)

One Post to Support the Heavens (Yi Zhu Ding Tian, 一柱頂天)

Play the Guitar (Shou Hui Pi Pa, 手揮琵琶)

Press Shoulder with Single Finger / Extending the Neck for Water (Yi Zhi Ding Jian / Yin Jing Qiu Shui, 一指頂肩 / 引頸求水)

Prop Up Elbow (Shang Jia Zhou, 上架肘)

Push the Boat to Follow the Stream (Shun Shui Tui Zhou, 順水推舟)

Repulse the Monkey (Dao Nian Hou, 倒撵猴)

Reverse Elbow Wrap (Fan Chan Zhou, 反纏肘)

Reverse Wrist Press (Fan Ya Wan, 反壓腕)

Roast Peking Duck (Bei Ping Kao Ya, 北平烤鴨)

Send the Devil to Heaven (Song Mo Shang Tian, 送魔上天)

Seven Stars to Lock the Throat (Qi Xing Suo Hou, 七星鎖喉)

Small Elbow Wrap (Xiao Chan Zhou, 小纏肘)

Small Wrap Finger (Xiao Chan Zhi, 小纏指)

Small Wrap Hand (Xiao Chan Shou, 小纏手)

Squeeze to Seal the Breath (Ji Xiong Bi Qi, 擠胸閉氣)

Step Forward and Deflect Downward (Shang Bu Ban Zhou, 上步扳肘)

Turn the Body to Seize the Monkey (Fan Shen Qin Yuan, 翻身擒猿)

Twist the Wrist and Push the Neck (Niu Wan Tui Jing, 扭腕推頸)

Twist the Wrist Under the Elbow (Zhou Di Zhi Wan, 肘底制腕)

Two Children Worship the Buddha (Shuang Tong Bai Fo, 雙童拜佛)

Two Hands Push the Chest (Shuang Shou Tui Xiong, 雙手推胸)

Two Hands Squeeze the Wrist (Shuang Shou Ji Wan, 雙手擠腕)

Upward Elbow Press (Shang Ya Zhou, 上壓肘)

Upward Elbow Wrap (Shang Chan Zhou, 上纏肘)

Upward Finger Turn (Shang Fen Zhi, 上分指)

Upward Pushing Enemy's Elbow (Shang Tui Di Zhou, 上推敵肘)

Upward Wrist Press (Shang Ya Wan, 上壓腕)

Upward, Horizontal, and Downward Wrist Press (Shang, Zhong, Xia Ya Wan, 上，中，下壓腕)

Use Both Hands to Lead the Cow (Shuang Shou Qian Niu, 雙手牽牛)

Wardoff Upward the Opponent's Elbow (Shang Peng Di Zhou, 上掤敵肘)

Wave Hands in Clouds (Yun Shou, 雲手)

White Crane Bores the Bush (Bai He Chuan Cong, 白鶴穿叢)

White Crane Covers Its Wings (Bai He Yan Chi, 白鶴掩翅)

White Crane Twists Its Neck (Bai He Niu Jing, 白鶴扭頸)

Wild Chicken Breaks Its Wings (Ye Ji Yao Chi, 野雞拗翅)

Wild Horses Shear the Mane (Ye Ma Fen Zong, 野馬分鬃)

Word "Ten" Pressing Leg (Shi Zi Ding Tui, 十字頂腿)

# Appendix B

## Translation of Thirty-Seven Postures

1. Grasp Sparrow's Tail (Lan Qiu Wei, 攬雀尾)
2. Wardoff (Peng, 掤)
3. Rollback (Lu, 攦)
4. Press or Squeeze (Ji, 擠)
5. Settle Down the Wrist (An, 按)
6. Single Whip (Dan Bian, 單鞭)
7. Lift Hands and Lean Forward (Ti Shou Shang Shi, 提手上勢)
8. Crane Spreads Its Wings (Bai He Liang Chi, 白鶴亮翅)
9. Brush Knee and Step Forward (Lou Xi Yao Bu, 摟膝拗步)
10. Play the Guitar (Shou Hui Pi Pa, 手揮琵琶)
11. Twist Body and Circle Fist (Pie Shen Chui, 撇身捶)
12. Step Forward, Deflect Downward, Parry, and Punch (Shang Bu Ban Lan Chui, 上步扳攔捶)
13. Seal Tightly (Ru Feng Si Bi, 如封似閉)
14. Embrace Tiger and Return to the Mountain (Bao Hu Gui Shan, 抱虎歸山)
15. Fist Under the Elbow (Zhou Di Kan Chui, 肘底看捶)
16. Step Back and Repulse Monkey (Dao Nian Hou, 倒攆猴)
17. Diagonal Flying (Xie Fei Shi, 斜飛勢)
18. Pick Up Needle from Sea Bottom (Hai Di Lao Zhen, 海底撈針)
19. Fan Back (Shan Tong Bei, 扇通背)
20. Wave Hands in Clouds (Yun Shou, 雲手)
21. Stand High to Search Out the Horse (Gao Tan Ma, 高探馬)
22. Toe Kick (Ti Tui, 踢腿)
23. Heel Kick (Deng Tui, 蹬腿)
24. Step Forward and Strike Down with the Fist (Jin Bu Zai Chui, 進步栽捶)
25. Strike the Tiger Posture (Da Hu Shi, 打虎勢)
26. Two Winds Pass Through the Ears (Shuang Feng Guan Er, 雙風貫耳)
27. Wild Horses Shear the Mane (Ye Ma Feng Zong, 野馬分鬃)

28.  Fair Lady Weaves with Shuttle (Yu Niu Chuan Suo, 玉女穿梭)

29.  Lower the Snake Body (She Shen Xia Shi, 蛇身下勢)

30.  Golden Rooster Stands on One Leg (Jin Ji Du Li, 金雞獨立)

31.  White Snake Turns Body and Spits Poison (Bai She Tu Xin, 白蛇吐信)

32.  Cross Hands (Shi Zi Shou, 十字手)

33.  Word "Ten" Leg (Shi Zi Tui, 十字腿)

34.  Step Forward to Seven Stars (Shang Bu Qi Xing, 上步七星)

35.  Step Back to Ride the Tiger (Tui Bu Kua Hu, 退步跨虎)

36.  Step Forward to Sweep Lotus (Shang Bu Bai Lian, 上步擺蓮)

37.  Draw the Bow and Shoot the Tiger (Wan Gong She Hu, 彎弓射虎)

# Appendix C

## Translation and Glossary of Chinese Terms

**aikido** (合氣道). A style of Japanese martial arts that uses the same theory of Chinese taijiquan and qin na.

**an** (按). Pressing or stamping. One of the eight basic taiji jing patterns.

**baguazhang** (八卦掌). Based on the eight trigrams palm, and found in the *Ye Jing*. One of the internal qigong martial styles believed to be created by Dong, Hai-chuan between AD 1866 and 1880.

**bai he** (白鶴). A Chinese southern martial style, called white crane.

**bei kao** (背靠). Using any part of the back to bump someone off balance.

**bi** (閉). Close or seal.

**bi qi** (閉氣). To seal the oxygen supply or close off the breath.

**cai** (採). To pluck.

**ce kao** (側靠). To bump someone off balance from the side.

**chai** (釵). Also called sai. A kind of hairpin for ancient Chinese women. Later it became a type of southern Chinese weapon.

**chan** (纏). To wrap or to coil. A common Chinese martial arts technique.

**chan jing** (纏勁). The martial power of wrapping or coiling.

**changquan** (長拳). Also called chang chuan. Includes all northern Chinese long-range martial styles. This term translates as long range fist and can refer to taijiquan.

**Chang, San-feng** (張三豐). Credited as the creator of taijiquan during the Song dynasty (宋代) (AD 960–1127) in China.

**Chang, Xiang-San** (張詳三). A well-known Chinese martial artist in Taiwan who was Mr. Wilson Chen's taijiquan master.

**Chen, Wilson** (陳威伸). Dr. Yang, Jwing-Ming's friend.

**Chen Style** (陳氏). The family of Chen.

**Chen, Yan-Lin** (陳炎林). A well-known taijiquan master in China during the 1940s.

**Cheng, Gin-Gsao** (曾金灶). Dr. Yang, Jwing-Ming's White Crane master.

**chi** (qi) (氣). The energy pervading the universe, including the energy circulating in the human body.

**chin** (qin) (擒). To catch or to seize.

**chin na** (qin na) (擒拿). A component of Chinese martial arts that emphasizes grabbing techniques to control your opponent's joints, in conjunction with attacking certain acupuncture cavities.

**cuo** (錯). To misplace or to disorder.

**cuo gu** (錯骨). Cuo means to disorder, and gu is bone. Therefore, cuo gu means to misplace the bone or joint.

**da** (打). To strike. Normally, to attack with the palms, fists, or arms.

**da lu** (大攦). Means "large rollback." One of the basic pushing hands practices in taiji-quan.

**Da Mo** (達摩). The Indian Buddhist monk who is credited with writing the *Yi Jin Jing* and *Xi Sui Jing* (易筋經，洗髓經) while at the Shaolin Monastery. His last name was Chadili, and he was also known as Bodhidharma. He was once the prince of a small tribe in southern India.

**da quan** (大圈). Large circle. One of the common fighting distances.

**da xue** (打穴). A category used in cavity striking.

**dabao** (Sp-21) (大包). An acupuncture cavity belonging to the spleen channel.

**dan tian** (丹田). Literally, field of elixir. Locations in the body that are able to store and generate qi (elixir) in the body. The upper, middle, and lower dan tian are located respectively between the eyebrows, at the solar plexus, and a few inches below the navel.

**Dao** (道). The "way," and by implication, the "natural way."

**dao** (倒). To turn over or reverse.

**dian** (點). To point or to press.

**dian mai** (點脈). Also called dim mak (Cantonese). Mai is the blood vessel (xue mai, 血脈) or the qi channel (qi mai, 氣脈). Dian mai means "to press the blood vessel or qi channel."

**dian xue** (點穴). Xue is the cavities. The term refers to qin na (擒拿) techniques that specialize in attacking acupuncture cavities to immobilize or kill an opponent.

**diao** (刁). Hooking.

**dim mak** (點脈). Cantonese of "dian mai."

**ding** (定). To stabilize or to firm.

**dong jing** (懂勁). "Understanding jing." A jing that uses the feeling of the skin to sense the opponent's energy.

**du mai** (督脈). Usually translated as governing vessel. One of the eight extraordinary vessels.

**duan** (斷). To break or to seal.

**duan mai** (斷脈). To seal or to break the blood vessel.

**dui** (兌). One of the eight trigrams.

**Emei** (峨嵋). Name of a mountain in Sichuan Province, China.

**ermen** (TB-21) (耳門). An acupuncture cavity belonging to the triple burner channel.

**fa jing** (發勁). Emitting jing. The power that is generally used for an attack.

**fen** (分). To divide.

**fen jin** (分筋). Means to divide the muscles/tendons (of your opponent).

**feng** (封). To seal or to cover.

**huo** (火). Fire, one of the five elements.

**futu** (LI-18) (伏兔). An acupuncture cavity belonging to the large intestine channel.

**gen** (艮). One of the eight trigrams.

**gongfu** (功夫). Also called kung fu. Energy-time. Anything that will take time and energy to learn or to accomplish is called gongfu.

**gu** (骨). Bone.

**guoshu** (國術). Abbreviation for "Zhongguo wushu" (中國武術), which means Chinese martial techniques. See also wushu.

**Han dynasty** (漢朝). A dynasty in Chinese history (206 BC–AD 221).

**Han, Ching-Tang** (韓慶堂). A well-known Chinese martial artist, especially in Taiwan. Master Han is also Dr. Yang, Jwing-Ming's Long Fist grand master.

**he** (合). Means to close.

**hou tian fa** (後天法). Post-heaven techniques, an internal qigong style dating from AD 550.

**hsing yi chuan** (形意拳) Also called xingyiquan. A style of internal Chinese martial arts.

**hua** (化). To neutralize.

**hua jing** (化勁). Neutralizing jing. Special taijiquan power training that allows you to neutralize incoming force.

**ji** (擠). To squeeze or to press.

**jiache** (S-6) (頰車). Name of an acupuncture cavity. It belongs to the stomach channel.

**jian kao** (肩靠). Shoulder bump. Refers to the use of the shoulder to bump someone off balance.

**jianjing** (GB-21) (肩井). An acupuncture cavity belonging to the gall bladder channel.

**jianneiling** (M-UE-48) (肩內陵). Name of an acupuncture cavity found midway between the underarm and the shoulder bone. A special point.

**jin** (筋). Means muscle/tendon.

**jing** (勁). In Chinese martial arts, it is the muscular power, li, which has been energized by qi to the maximum potential.

**jin bu** (進步). Step forward. Taijiquan is constructed from thirteen basic postures, which include basic moving patterns and strategic steppings. Jin bu is one of the five steppings.

**Jin, Shao-Feng** (金紹峰). Dr. Yang, Jwing-Ming's White Crane grandmaster.

**jiquan** (H-1) (極泉). An acupuncture cavity belonging to the heart channel.

**jiuwei** (Co-15) (鳩尾). An acupuncture cavity belonging to the conception vessel.

**Jou, Tsung-Hwa** (AD 1917–1998) (周宗樺). A well-known taijiquan master in America.

**judo** (柔道). A style of Japanese martial arts similar to wrestling.

**jujitsu** (柔術道). A style of Japanese martial arts that uses theories similar to Chinese taijiquan and qin na.

**kan** (坎). One of the eight trigrams.

**kao** (靠). Means "bump." One of the taijiquan thirteen postures.

**kong qi** (空氣). Air.

**kun** (坤). One of the eight trigrams.

**li** (離). A phase of the eight trigrams (bagua, 八卦), li represents fire.

**Li, Mao-Ching** (李茂清). Dr. Yang, Jwing-Ming's Long Fist master.

**Liang dynasty** (梁朝). A dynasty in Chinese history (AD 502–557).

**Liang, Dexing** (Jeffrey D. S. Liang) (梁德馨). Master Liang, Shou-Yu's uncle. Dexing Liang currently residing in Seattle, Washington.

**Liang, Shou-Yu** (梁守渝). A well-known Chinese martial arts and qigong master who currently resides in Vancouver, Canada.

**Liang Wu** (梁武). An emperor of the Chinese Liang dynasty.

**lie** (挒). Split or rend. One of the thirteen basic postures in taijiquan.

**lie jing** (挒勁). The martial power of rend.

**lien bu chuan** (連步拳). One of the long fist bare hand sequences.

**lingtai** (Gv-10) (靈台). Spiritual station. An acupuncture cavity located on the governing vessel (du mai, 督脈).

**liu he ba fa** (六合八法). Literally, "six combinations eight methods." One of the Chinese internal martial arts, its techniques are combined from taijiquan (太極拳), xingyiquan (形意拳), and baguazhang (八卦掌). This internal martial art was reportedly created by Chen, Bo (陳博) during the Song dynasty (宋代) (AD 960–1279).

**lu** (掤). Rollback. One of the thirteen basic postures in taijiquan.

**mai** (脈). Means vessel or qi channel.

**mu** (木). Wood. One of the five elements.

**na** (拿). To hold or to grab. Also an abbreviation for chin na or qin na.

**na xue** (拿穴). To grab the cavity.

**na xue** (拿血). To grab the blood vessel.

**naohu** (Gv-17, 腦戶). An acupuncture cavity belonging to the governing vessel.

**Nanking Central Guoshu Institute** (南京中央國術館). A national martial arts institute organized by the Chinese government in 1926.

**neiguan** (P-6) (內關). An acupuncture cavity belonging to the pericardium channel.

**pao chui** (炮捶). The second routine of Chen Style Taijiquan.

**peng** (掤). Wardoff. One of the taijiquan basic thirteen postures.

**peng jing** (掤勁). The martial power of wardoff.

**peng kai** (掤開). Push open. Peng means to arc your arms and use them to push or bounce your opponent away.

**qi** (chi) (氣). The general definition of qi is universal energy, including heat, light, and electromagnetic energy. A narrower definition of qi refers to the energy circulating in human or animal bodies. A current popular model is that the qi circulating in the human body is bioelectric in nature.

**qi chen dan tian** (氣沉丹田). "Sink the qi to the lower dan tian." The name of a taijiquan posture.

**qi mai** (氣脈). Means qi channels.

**qian** (乾). One of the eight trigrams.

**qian kao** (前靠). Forward bump. To bump someone off balance from his front.

**qigong** (氣功). Also called chi kung. Gong means energy-time. Therefore, qigong means study, research, and practices related to qi.

**qihai** (Co-6) (氣海). An acupuncture cavity belonging to the conception vessel.

**qimen** (Li-14) (期門). An acupuncture cavity belonging to the liver channel.

**qin** (chin) (擒). To catch or to seize.

**qin na** (chin na) (擒拿). Called "grab control," a component of Chinese martial arts that emphasizes grabbing techniques to control your opponent's joints, in conjunction with attacking certain acupuncture cavities.

**qin xiong** (擒凶). To catch the murderer.

**quchi** (LI-11) (曲池). Name of an acupuncture cavity. It belongs to the large intestine channel.

**ren mai** (任脈). Conception vessel. One of the eight extraordinary vessels.

**renzhong** (Gv-26) (人中). An acupuncture cavity belonging to the governing vessel.

**riyue** (GB-24) (日月). An acupuncture cavity belonging to the gall bladder channel.

**rugen** (S-18) (乳根). An acupuncture cavity belonging to the stomach channel.

**ruzhong** (S-17) (乳中). An acupuncture cavity belonging to the stomach channel.

**sai** (chai) (釵). A kind of hairpin for ancient Chinese women. Later it was developed into a kind of southern Chinese weapon.

**san shi qi shi** (三十七勢). Thirty-seven postures. According to historical records, one of the predecessors of taijiquan.

**shang kao** (上靠). To lean or to press upward.

**shangen** (M-HN-4) (山根). An acupuncture cavity. A special point.

**shaohai** (H-3) (少海). Name of an acupuncture cavity. It belongs to the heart channel.

**Shaolin** (少林). "Young Woods." Name of the Shaolin Temple.

**Shaolin Temple** (少林寺). A monastery located in Henan Province (河南省), China. The Shaolin Temple is well known because of its martial arts training.

**shi san shi** (十三勢). Thirteen postures. Taijiquan is also called thirteen postures because it is constructed from thirteen basic moving patterns.

**shuai** (摔). To throw. It is a short-form reference to shuai jiao (wrestling).

**shuai jiao** (摔交). Chinese wrestling. Part of Chinese martial arts.

**Song dynasty** (宋朝). A dynasty in Chinese history (AD 960–1279).

**shui** (水). Water. One of the five elements.

**Sun** (孫). A last name of a Chinese family.

**Sun, Lu-Tang** (AD 1861–1932) (孫祿堂). A well-known martial artist in the early 1920s. He mastered many styles, such as baguazhang, xingyiquan, and taijiquan. He is also the creator of Sun Style Taijiquan.

**tai chi chuan** (taijiquan) (太極拳). A Chinese internal martial style based on the theory of taiji (grand ultimate).

**taiji** (太極). Means grand ultimate. It is the force that generates two poles, yin and yang.

**taiji huan yuan** (太極還原). Return taiji to its origin, which is the name of a taijiquan posture.

**taiji qi shi** (太極起勢). Taiji beginning, which is the name of a taijiquan posture.

**taijiquan** (tai chi chuan) (太極拳). A Chinese internal martial style based on the theory of taiji (grand ultimate).

**Taipei** (台北). The capital city of Taiwan, located in the north.

**Taipei Xian** (台北縣). The county in the north of Taiwan where Dr. Yang attended Tamkang College.

**Taiwan** (台灣). An island to the southeast of mainland China. Also known as Formosa.

**Taiwan University** (台灣大學). A well-known university located in northern Taiwan.

**taiyang** (M-HN-9) (太陽). Name of an acupuncture cavity found at the temple.

**taizuquan** (太祖拳). A style of Chinese external martial arts.

**Tamkang** (淡江). Name of a university in Taiwan.

**Tamkang College Guoshu Club** (淡江國術社). A Chinese martial arts club founded by Dr. Yang when he was studying in Tamkang College.

**Kao Tao** (高濤). Dr. Yang, Jwing-Ming's first taijiquan master.

**ti** (踢). To kick.

**ti** (提). To lift.

**tiantu** (Co-22) (天突). Name of an acupuncture cavity. It belongs to the conception vessel.

**tianrong** (SI-17) (天容). Name of an acupuncture cavity that belongs to the small intestine channel.

**tianzong** (SI-11) (天宗). Name of an acupuncture cavity. It belongs to the small intestine channel.

**ting jing** (聽勁). Listening jing. Special training in taijiquan that uses the feeling, especially the skin's sensitivity, to determine the opponent's intention.

**tu** (土). Earth. One of the five elements.

**tui bu** (退步). Step backward. One of the taijiquan thirteen postures. Taijiquan is constructed from eight basic moving patterns (eight doors) and five strategic steppings (five steppings). Tui bu is one of the five steppings.

**tui kao** (腿靠). Leg bump. Use the thigh to bump someone off balance.

**tui na** (推拿). A category of Chinese massages for healing and injury treatment.

**tun kao** (臀靠). Hip bump. To use the hip to bump someone off balance.

**wai dan chi kung** (外丹氣功). Same as wai dan qigong. External elixir qigong. In wai dan qigong, a practitioner will generate qi to the limbs and then allow the qi to flow inward to nourish the internal organs.

**Wang, Shu-tian** (王樹田). A well-known Chinese martial arts master.

**Wu** (吳). The last name of a Chinese family.

**wuji** (無極). Means no extremity. When motivated by action from taiji, becomes yin and yang.

**wushu** (武術). Literally, "martial techniques." A common name for the Chinese martial arts. Many other terms are used, including martial arts (wuyi, 武藝), martial gongfu (wugong, 武功), national techniques (guoshu, 國術), and energy-time (gongfu, 功夫). Because wushu has been modified in mainland China over the past forty years into gymnastic martial performances, many traditional Chinese martial artists have given up this name in order to avoid confusing modern wushu with traditional wushu. Recently, mainland China has attempted to bring modern wushu back toward its traditional training and practice.

**wuyi** (武藝). Another name for Chinese martial arts.

**xi kao** (膝靠). Knee bump, which is used to bump someone off balance.

**xia kao** (下靠). Downward bump. To bump someone off balance through a downward bumping action.

**xiao jiu tian** (小九天). Small nine heaven is a qigong style created in the sixth century.

**xiao lu** (小攦). Small rollback, a taijiquan pushing hands technique.

**xiao quan** (小圈). Small circle.

**xin** (心). The mind generated from emotional disturbance.

**xingyi** (形意). An abbreviation of xingyiquan.

**xingyiquan** (hsing yi chuan) (形意拳). Shape mind fist, an internal style of gongfu in which the mind or thinking determines the shape or movement of the body. Creation of the style is attributed to Marshal Yue, Fei (岳飛).

**Xinzhu Xian** (新竹縣). Birthplace of Dr. Yang, Jwing-Ming, in Taiwan.

**xiong kao** (胸靠). Chest bump. Use the chest to bump someone off balance.

**xue mai** (血脈). Means "blood vessels."

**xun** (巽). One of the eight trigrams.

**yang** (陽). In Chinese philosophy, the active, positive, masculine polarity. In Chinese medicine, yang means excessive, overactive, overheated. The yang (or outer) organs are the gall bladder, small intestine, large intestine, stomach, bladder, and triple burner.

**Yang, Jwing-Ming** (楊俊敏). Author of this book.

**Yang, Mei-Ling** (楊美玲). Master Yang, Jwing-Ming's wife.

**Yang Style** (楊氏). The style created by the Yang family.

**yi** (意). The mind that is generated by clear thinking and judgment, and that is able to make you calm, peaceful, and wise.

**yifeng** (TB-17) (翳風). Name of an acupuncture cavity. It belongs to the triple burner channel.

**yin** (陰). In Chinese philosophy, the passive, negative, feminine polarity. In Chinese medicine, yin means deficient. The yin (internal) organs are the heart, lungs, liver, kidneys, spleen, and pericardium.

**yin jing** (引勁). Leading jing. A special power that can lead the opponent's incoming force in a desired direction.

**yin qi gui yuan** (引氣歸原). Lead the qi to return to its origin, which is the name of a taijiquan posture.

**yingchuang** (S-16) (膺窗). Name of an acupuncture cavity. It belongs to the stomach channel.

**you pan** (右盼). Look to the right, one of the taijiquan thirteen postures.

**yuanye** (GB-22) (淵腋). Name of an acupuncture cavity. It belongs to the gall bladder channel.

**yun shou** (雲手). Wave hands in clouds, which is the name of a taijiquan posture.

**zhen** (震). One of the eight trigrams.

**zhong** (中). Centering.

**zhong ding** (中定). Firm the center, which is one of the taijiquan thirteen postures.

**zhong quan** (中圈). Middle circle.

**zhongwan** (Co-12) (中脘). Name of an acupuncture cavity. It belongs to the conception vessel.

**zhou** (肘). Elbow. Use the elbow to execute defensive or offensive techniques in taijiquan.

**zhua** (抓). To grasp or to grab.

**zhua jin** (抓筋). To grab the tendons.

**zhua xue** (抓穴). To grab the cavity.

**zhuan** (轉). To turn around or to twist.

**zi wu liu zhu** (子午流注). Zi refers to the period around midnight (11:00 p.m.–1:00 a.m.), and wu refers to midday (11:00 a.m.–1:00 p.m.). Jiu zhu means the flowing tendency. Incorporating this schedule of the qi circulation will show you the channel that has the predominant qi flow at any particular time, and where the predominant qi flow is in the conception and governing vessels.

**zuo** (左). Left.

**zuo gu** (左顧). Look to the left, one of the taijiquan thirteen postures.

**zuo wan** (坐腕). Settling the wrist occurs when the taijiquan practitioner uses the palm to strike; right before contact, the wrist is settled to firm the posture and alignment of the palm.

# Index

# About the Author

## Yang, Jwing-Ming, PhD (楊俊敏博士)

Dr. Yang, Jwing-Ming was born on August 11, 1946, in Xinzhu Xian (新竹縣), Taiwan (台灣), Republic of China (中華民國). He started his *wushu* (武術) (*gongfu* or *kung fu*, 功夫) training at the age of fifteen under Shaolin White Crane (Shaolin Bai He, 少林白鶴) Master, Cheng, Gin-Gsao (曾金灶). Master Cheng originally learned Taizuquan (太祖拳) from his grandfather when he was a child. When Master Cheng was fifteen years old, he started learning White Crane from Master Jin, Shao-Feng (金紹峰) and followed him for twenty-three years until Master Jin's death.

In thirteen years of study (1961–1974) under Master Cheng, Dr. Yang became an expert in the White Crane style of Chinese martial arts, which includes both the use of bare hand and various weapons, such as saber, staff, spear, trident, two short rods, and many other weapons. With the same master, he also studied White Crane Qigong (氣功), *qin na* or *chin na* (擒拿), *tui na* (推拿), and *dian xue* massages (點穴按摩) and herbal treatment.

At sixteen, Dr. Yang began the study of Yang Style Taijiquan (楊氏太極拳) under Master Kao Tao (高濤). He later continued his study of *taijiquan* under Master Li, Mao-Ching (李茂清), and also practiced with Mr. Wilson Chen (陳威伸), in Taipei (台北). Master Li learned his taijiquan from the well-known Master Han, Ching-Tang (韓慶堂), and Mr. Chen learned his taijiquan from Master Chang, Xiang-San (張詳三). From this further practice, Dr. Yang was able to master the *taiji* bare hand sequence, pushing hands, the two-man fighting sequence, taiji sword, taiji saber, and taiji qigong.

When Dr. Yang was eighteen years old, he entered Tamkang College (淡江學院) in Taipei Xian to study physics. In college, he began the study of traditional Shaolin Long Fist (*Changquan* or *Chang Chuan*, 少林長拳) with Master Li, Mao-Ching at the Tamkang College Guoshu Club (淡江國術社), 1964–1968, and eventually became an assistant instructor under Master Li. In 1971, he completed his MS degree in physics at the National Taiwan University (台灣大學) and then served in the Chinese Air Force from 1971 to 1972. In the service, Dr. Yang taught physics at the Junior Academy of the Chinese Air Force (空軍幼校) while also teaching wushu. After being honorably discharged in 1972, he returned to Tamkang College to teach physics and resumed study under Master Li, Mao-Ching. From Master Li, Dr. Yang learned Northern style wushu, which includes both bare hand and kicking techniques, and numerous weapons.

In 1974, Dr. Yang came to the United States to study mechanical engineering at Purdue University. At the request of a few students, Dr. Yang began to teach gongfu (kung fu), which resulted in the establishment of the Purdue University Chinese Kung Fu Research Club in the spring of 1975. While at Purdue, Dr. Yang also taught college-credit courses in taijiquan. In May of 1978, he was awarded a PhD in mechanical engineering by Purdue.

In 1980, Dr. Yang moved to Houston to work for Texas Instruments. While in Houston, he founded Yang's Shaolin Kung Fu Academy, which was eventually taken over by his disciple, Mr. Jeffery Bolt, after Dr. Yang moved to Boston in 1982. Dr. Yang founded Yang's Martial Arts Academy in Boston on October 1, 1982.

In January of 1984, he gave up his engineering career to devote more time to research, writing, and teaching. In March of 1986, he purchased property in the Jamaica Plain area of Boston to be used as the headquarters of the new organization, Yang's Martial Arts Association (YMAA). The organization expanded to become a division of Yang's Oriental Arts Association, Inc. (YOAA).

In 2008, Dr. Yang began the nonprofit YMAA California Retreat Center. This training facility in rural California is where selected students enroll in a five-year residency to learn Chinese martial arts.

Dr. Yang has been involved in traditional Chinese wushu since 1961, studying Shaolin White Crane (*Bai He*), Shaolin Long Fist (*Changquan*), and taijiquan under several different masters. He has taught for more than forty-six years: seven years in Taiwan, five years at Purdue University, two years in Houston, twenty-six years in Boston, and six years at the YMAA California Retreat Center. He has taught seminars all around the world, sharing his knowledge of Chinese martial arts and qigong in Argentina, Austria, Barbados, Botswana, Belgium, Bermuda, Brazil, Canada, China, Chile, England, Egypt, France, Germany, Holland, Hungary, Iceland, Iran, Ireland, Italy, Latvia, Mexico, New Zealand, Poland, Portugal, Saudi Arabia, Spain, South Africa, Switzerland, and Venezuela.

Since 1986, YMAA has become an international organization, which currently includes more than fifty schools located in Argentina, Belgium, Canada, Chile, France, Hungary, Iran, Ireland, Italy, New Zealand, Poland, Portugal, South Africa, Sweden, the United Kingdom, Venezuela, and the United States.

Many of Dr. Yang's books and videos have been translated into languages, such as French, Italian, Spanish, Polish, Czech, Bulgarian, Russian, German, and Hungarian.

## Books and Videos by Dr. Yang, Jwing-Ming

Books Alphabetical

*Analysis of Shaolin Chin Na,* 2nd ed. YMAA Publication Center, 1987, 2004

*Ancient Chinese Weapons: A Martial Artist's Guide,* 2nd ed. YMAA Publication Center, 1985, 1999

*Arthritis Relief: Chinese Qigong for Healing & Prevention,* 2nd ed. YMAA Publication Center, 1991, 2005

*Back Pain Relief: Chinese Qigong for Healing and Prevention,* 2nd ed. YMAA Publication Center, 1997, 2004

*Baguazhang: Theory and Applications,* 2nd ed. YMAA Publication Center, 1994, 2008

*Comprehensive Applications of Shaolin Chin Na: The Practical Defense of Chinese Seizing Arts.* YMAA Publication Center, 1995

*How to Defend Yourself.* YMAA Publication Center, 1992

*Introduction to Ancient Chinese Weapons.* Unique Publications, Inc., 1985

*Northern Shaolin Sword,* 2nd ed. YMAA Publication Center, 1985, 2000

*Qigong for Health and Martial Arts*, 2nd ed. YMAA Publication Center, 1995, 1998

*Qigong Massage: Fundamental Techniques for Health and Relaxation,* 2nd ed. YMAA Publication Center, 1992, 2005

*Qigong Meditation: Embryonic Breathing.* YMAA Publication Center, 2003

*Qigong Meditation: Small Circulation.* YMAA Publication Center, 2006

*Qigong, the Secret of Youth: Da Mo's Muscle/Tendon Changing and Marrow/Brain Washing Qigong,* 2nd ed. YMAA Publication Center, 1989, 2000

*Shaolin Chin Na.* Unique Publications, Inc., 1980

*Shaolin Long Fist Kung Fu.* Unique Publications, Inc., 1981

*Simple Qigong Exercises for Health: The Eight Pieces of Brocade,* 3rd ed. YMAA Publication Center, 1988, 1997, 2013

*Tai Chi Ball Qigong: For Health and Martial Arts.* YMAA Publication Center, 2010

*Tai Chi Chuan Classical Yang Style: The Complete Long Form and Qigong,* 2nd ed. YMAA Publication Center, 1999, 2010

*Tai Chi Chuan Martial Applications*, 2nd ed. YMAA Publication Center, 1986, 1996

*Tai Chi Chuan: Classical Yang Style,* 2nd ed. YMAA Publication Center, 1999, 2010

*Tai Chi Qigong: The Internal Foundation of Tai Chi Chuan,* 2nd ed., rev. YMAA Publication Center, 1997, 1990, 2013

*Tai Chi Secrets of the Ancient Masters: Selected Readings with Commentary.* YMAA Publication Center, 1999

*Tai Chi Secrets of the Wŭ and Li Styles: Chinese Classics, Translation, Commentary.* YMAA Publication Center, 2001

*Tai Chi Secrets of the Wu Style: Chinese Classics, Translation, Commentary.* YMAA Publication Center, 2002

*Tai Chi Secrets of the Yang Style: Chinese Classics, Translation, Commentary.* YMAA Publication Center, 2001

*Tai Chi Sword Classical Yang Style: The Complete Long Form, Qigong, and Applications,* 2nd ed. YMAA Publication Center, 1999, 2014

*Tai Chi Theory and Martial Power,* 2nd ed. YMAA Publication Center, 1986, 1996

*Taiji Chin Na: The Seizing Art of Taijiquan.* YMAA Publication Center, 1995

*Taijiquan Theory of Dr. Yang, Jwing-Ming: The Root of Taijiquan.* YMAA Publication Center, 2003

*The Essence of Shaolin White Crane.* YMAA Publication Center, 1996

*The Root of Chinese Qigong: The Secrets of Qigong Training,* 2nd ed. YMAA Publication Center, 1989, 2004

*Xingyiquan: Theory and Applications,* 2nd ed. YMAA Publication Center, 1990, 2003

*Yang Style Tai Chi Chuan.* Unique Publications, Inc., 1981


Videos Alphabetical

*Advanced Practical Chin Na In Depth.* YMAA Publication Center, 2010

*Analysis of Shaolin Chin Na.* YMAA Publication Center, 2004

*Baguazhang (Eight Trigrams Palm Kung Fu).* YMAA Publication Center, 2005

*Chin Na In Depth: Courses 1–4.* YMAA Publication Center, 2003

*Chin Na In Depth: Courses 5–8.* YMAA Publication Center, 2003

*Chin Na In Depth: Courses 9–12.* YMAA Publication Center, 2003

*Five Animal Sports Qigong.* YMAA Publication Center, 2008

*Knife Defense: Traditional Techniques.* YMAA Publication Center, 2011

*Meridian Qigong: Combined Qigong, Yoga, and Acupuncture Exercises.* YMAA Publication Center, 2014

*Northern Shaolin Sword.* YMAA Publication Center, 2009

*Qigong Massage.* YMAA Publication Center, 2005

*Saber Fundamental Training.* YMAA Publication Center, 2008

*Shaolin Kung Fu Fundamental Training.* YMAA Publication Center, 2004

*Shaolin Long Fist Kung Fu: Basic Sequences.* YMAA Publication Center, 2005

*Shaolin Saber Basic Sequences.* YMAA Publication Center, 2007

*Shaolin Staff Basic Sequences.* YMAA Publication Center, 2007

*Shaolin White Crane Gong Fu Basic Training: Courses 1 & 2.* YMAA Publication Center, 2003

*Shaolin White Crane Gong Fu Basic Training: Courses 3 & 4.* YMAA Publication Center, 2008

*Shaolin White Crane Hard and Soft Qigong.* YMAA Publication Center, 2003

*Shuai Jiao: Kung Fu Wrestling.* YMAA Publication Center, 2010

*Simple Qigong Exercises for Arthritis Relief.* YMAA Publication Center, 2007

*Simple Qigong Exercises for Back Pain Relief.* YMAA Publication Center, 2007

*Simple Qigong Exercises for Health: The Eight Pieces of Brocade.* YMAA Publication Center, 2003

*Staff Fundamental Training: Solo Drills and Matching Practice.* YMAA Publication Center, 2007

*Sword Fundamental Training.* YMAA Publication Center, 2009

*Tai Chi Ball Qigong: Courses 1 & 2.* YMAA Publication Center, 2006

*Tai Chi Ball Qigong: Courses 3 & 4.* YMAA Publication Center, 2007

*Tai Chi Chuan: Classical Yang Style.* YMAA Publication Center, 2003

*Tai Chi Fighting Set: 2-Person Matching Set. YMAA Publication Center, 2006*

*Tai Chi Pushing Hands: Courses 1 & 2.* YMAA Publication Center, 2005

*Tai Chi Pushing Hands: Courses 3 & 4.* YMAA Publication Center, 2006

*Tai Chi Qigong.* YMAA Publication Center, 2005

*Tai Chi Sword, Classical Yang Style.* YMAA Publication Center, 2005

*Tai Chi Symbol: Yin/Yang Sticking Hands.* YMAA Publication Center, 2008

*Taiji 37 Postures Martial Applications.* YMAA Publication Center, 2008

*Taiji Chin Na in Depth.* YMAA Publication Center, 2009

*Taiji Saber: Classical Yang Style.* YMAA Publication Center, 2008

*Taiji Wrestling: Advanced Takedown Techniques.* YMAA Publication Center, 2008

*Understanding Qigong, DVD 1: What is Qigong? The Human Qi Circulatory System.* YMAA Publication Center, 2006

*Understanding Qigong, DVD 2: Key Points of Qigong & Qigong Breathing.* YMAA Publication Center, 2006

*Understanding Qigong, DVD 3: Embryonic Breathing.* YMAA Publication Center, 2007

*Understanding Qigong, DVD 4: Four Seasons Qigong.* YMAA Publication Center, 2007

*Understanding Qigong, DVD 5: Small Circulation.* YMAA Publication Center, 2007

*Understanding Qigong, DVD 6: Martial Arts Qigong Breathing.* YMAA Publication Center, 2007

*Xingyiquan: Twelve Animals Kung Fu and Applications.* YMAA Publication Center, 2008

*Yang Tai Chi for Beginners.* YMAA Publication Center, 2012

*YMAA 25-Year Anniversary.* YMAA Publication Center, 2009

## BOOKS FROM YMAA

6 HEALING MOVEMENTS
101 REFLECTIONS ON TAI CHI CHUAN
108 INSIGHTS INTO TAI CHI CHUAN
ADVANCING IN TAE KWON DO
ANALYSIS OF SHAOLIN CHIN NA 2ND ED
ANCIENT CHINESE WEAPONS
ART OF HOJO UNDO
ARTHRITIS RELIEF, 3RD ED.
BACK PAIN RELIEF, 2ND ED.
BAGUAZHANG, 2ND ED.
CARDIO KICKBOXING ELITE
CHIN NA IN GROUND FIGHTING
CHINESE FAST WRESTLING
CHINESE FITNESS
CHINESE TUI NA MASSAGE
CHOJUN
COMPREHENSIVE APPLICATIONS OF SHAOLIN
    CHIN NA
CROCODILE AND THE CRANE: A NOVEL
CUTTING SEASON: A XENON PEARL MARTIAL
    ARTS THRILLER
DESHI: A CONNOR BURKE MARTIAL ARTS THRILLER
DIRTY GROUND
DR. WU'S HEAD MASSAGE
DUKKHA REVERB
DUKKHA, THE SUFFERING: AN EYE FOR AN EYE
DUKKHA UNLOADED
ENZAN: THE FAR MOUNTAIN, A CONNOR BURKE MARTIAL
    ARTS THRILLER
ESSENCE OF SHAOLIN WHITE CRANE
EXPLORING TAI CHI
FACING VIOLENCE
FIGHTING ARTS
FORCE DECISIONS: A CITIZENS GUIDE
FOX BORROWS THE TIGER'S AWE
INSIDE TAI CHI
KAGE: THE SHADOW, A CONNOR BURKE MARTIAL ARTS
    THRILLER
KATA AND THE TRANSMISSION OF KNOWLEDGE
KRAV MAGA: WEAPON DEFENSES
LITTLE BLACK BOOK OF VIOLENCE
LIUHEBAFA FIVE CHARACTER SECRETS
MARTIAL ARTS ATHLETE
MARTIAL ARTS INSTRUCTION
MARTIAL WAY AND ITS VIRTUES
MASK OF THE KING
MEDITATIONS ON VIOLENCE
MIND/BODY FITNESS
MUGAI RYU
NATURAL HEALING WITH QIGONG
NORTHERN SHAOLIN SWORD, 2ND ED.
OKINAWA'S COMPLETE KARATE SYSTEM: ISSHIN RYU
POWER BODY
PRINCIPLES OF TRADITIONAL CHINESE MEDICINE
QIGONG FOR HEALTH & MARTIAL ARTS 2ND ED.
QIGONG FOR LIVING
QIGONG FOR TREATING COMMON AILMENTS

QIGONG MASSAGE
QIGONG MEDITATION: EMBRYONIC BREATHING
QIGONG MEDITATION: SMALL CIRCULATION
QIGONG, THE SECRET OF YOUTH: DA MO'S CLASSICS
QUIET TEACHER: A XENON PEARL MARTIAL ARTS THRILLER
RAVEN'S WARRIOR
ROOT OF CHINESE QIGONG, 2ND ED.
SCALING FORCE
SENSEI: A CONNOR BURKE MARTIAL ARTS THRILLER
SHIHAN TE: THE BUNKAI OF KATA
SHIN GI TAI: KARATE TRAINING FOR BODY, MIND, AND
    SPIRIT
SIMPLE CHINESE MEDICINE
SIMPLE QIGONG EXERCISES FOR HEALTH, 3RD ED.
SIMPLIFIED TAI CHI CHUAN, 3RD ED.
SUDDEN DAWN: THE EPIC JOURNEY OF BODHIDHARMA
SUNRISE TAI CHI
SUNSET TAI CHI
SURVIVING ARMED ASSAULTS
TAE KWON DO: THE KOREAN MARTIAL ART
TAEKWONDO BLACK BELT POOMSAE
TAEKWONDO: A PATH TO EXCELLENCE
TAEKWONDO: ANCIENT WISDOM FOR THE MODERN
    WARRIOR
TAEKWONDO: DEFENSES AGAINST WEAPONS
TAEKWONDO: SPIRIT AND PRACTICE
TAO OF BIOENERGETICS
TAI CHI BALL QIGONG: FOR HEALTH AND MARTIAL ARTS
TAI CHI BOOK
TAI CHI CHIN NA: THE SEIZING ART OF TAI CHI CHUAN
TAI CHI CHUAN CLASSICAL YANG STYLE (REVISED
    EDITION)
TAI CHI CHUAN MARTIAL APPLICATIONS, 2ND ED.
TAI CHI CONNECTIONS
TAI CHI DYNAMICS
TAI CHI QIGONG, 3RD ED.
TAI CHI SECRETS OF THE ANCIENT MASTERS
TAI CHI SECRETS OF THE WU & LI STYLES
TAI CHI SECRETS OF THE WU STYLE
TAI CHI SECRETS OF THE YANG STYLE
TAI CHI SWORD: CLASSICAL YANG STYLE
TAI CHI THEORY & MARTIAL POWER, 2ND ED.
TAI CHI WALKING
TAIJIQUAN THEORY OF DR. YANG, JWING-MING
TENGU: THE MOUNTAIN GOBLIN, A CONNOR BURKE
    MARTIAL ARTS THRILLER
TRADITIONAL CHINESE HEALTH SECRETS
TRADITIONAL TAEKWONDO
WAY OF KATA
WAY OF KENDO AND KENJITSU
WAY OF SANCHIN KATA
WAY TO BLACK BELT
WESTERN HERBS FOR MARTIAL ARTISTS
WILD GOOSE QIGONG
WISDOM'S WAY
WOMAN'S QIGONG GUIDE
XINGYIQUAN, 2ND ED.

*continued on next page . . .*

## DVDS FROM YMAA

*more products available from . . .*

**YMAA Publication Center, Inc.** 楊氏東方文化出版中心

1-800-669-8892 • info@ymaa.com • www.ymaa.com